Sober

*The Most Effective Guide on How to
Achieve Sobriety, Ridding Oneself of
Alcoholism, and Learning to Rebuild a
Life of Wellness, Alcohol-Free*

Richard Banks

© Copyright 2021 by Richard Banks. All right reserved
The content contained within this book may not be reproduced, duplicated or transmitted without direct written permission from the author or the publisher.

Under no circumstances will any blame or legal responsibility be held against the publisher, or author, for any damages, reparation, or monetary loss due to the information contained within this book. Either directly or indirectly.

Legal Notice:

This book is copyright protected. This book is only for personal use. You cannot amend, distribute, sell, use, quote or paraphrase any part, or the content within this book, without the consent of the author or publisher.

Disclaimer Notice:

Please note the information contained within this document is for educational and entertainment purposes only. All effort has been executed to present accurate, up to date, and reliable, complete information. No warranties of any kind are declared or implied. Readers acknowledge that the author is not engaging in the rendering of legal, financial, medical or professional advice. The content within this book has been derived from various sources. Please consult a licensed professional before attempting any techniques outlined in this book.

By reading this document, the reader agrees that under no circumstances is the author responsible for any losses, direct or indirect, which are incurred as a result of the use of the information contained within this document, including, but not limited to, — errors, omissions, or inaccuracies.

Thank You!

Thank you for your purchase.

I am dedicated to making the most enriching and informational content. I hope it meets your expectations and you gain a lot from it.

Your comments and feedback are important to me because they help me to provide the best material possible. So, if you have any questions or concerns, please email me at richardbanks.books@gmail.com.

Again, thank you for your purchase.

Introduction 7

Chapter 1 - Alcohol in Our Culture 15

The Alcohol Illusion 20

What Is Alcoholism? 23

What Is an Alcoholic? 26

Chapter 2 - Understanding Your Habits and Needs 33

The Basics of Habits 33

Your Most Fundamental Needs 34

Understanding Why You Drink 38

What Does it Mean to Stop Drinking Alcohol? 44

Recognizing You Have a Problem 45

Hitting Rock Bottom 52

Sobriety 55

Chapter 3 – First Steps to Freedom 59

Professional Help and Support 59

Expectations 62

Mindset 64

Preparation 65

Detox and Withdrawal 76

Chapter 4 – The Approach 81

Principle 1: Addiction 82

Principle 2: Biological 87

Principle 3: Psychological 87

Principle 4: Social 88

Chapter 5 – Addiction Focus 91

A Brief History of Addiction 91

The Addiction Cycle 93

Recognizing Relapse Warning Signs 99

Chapter 6 – Biological Focus 103

Nutrition 104

Fitness and Exercise 109

Sleep 110

Fueling Your Body's Capacity to Heal 112

Chapter 7 – Psychological Focus 115

Mastering Your Mental Health 115

Chapter 8 – Social Focus 129

Family and Friends 130

Professional Relationships 132

Seek Support from Safe People 134

Chapter 9 – Sobriety Success 137

Conclusion 143

Bonus Chapter 149

Books by Richard Banks 179

Introduction

"Sometimes we motivate ourselves by thinking of what we want to become. And sometimes we motivate ourselves by thinking about who we don't ever want to be again." – Shane Niemeyer

From suicides to homicides to traffic accidents, the infamous beverage has played the starring role in more than half of accidental and deliberate deaths in the United States, rounding up to 95,000 a year as we speak. If we narrow that down, we find that one in 12 adults in the USA regularly uses alcohol. The National Institute of Alcohol Abuse & Alcoholism deems it the third-leading preventable cause of death in America, citing that it's the main culprit in four out of 10 fatal accidents, falls, and automobile crashes. As a contributor to liver cirrhosis, various kinds of cancer, high blood pressure, sexual dysfunction, and more, alcohol is a silent killer that manifests its effects on not just your physical body but in your personal and professional life as well.

The sedative effects of alcohol contribute to its widespread consumption. While it does help numb the emotional pain of the person who indulges, it may also be the very cause of that pain. Drinking to escape your problems or overindulging for the thrill of getting drunk can have lifelong repercussions. Broken relationships, toppling careers, and deteriorating health are only the beginning. From a swollen abdomen to slipping into a coma, the effects of alcohol can be fatal, and denying its dangers will only prolong your path to recovery.

Quitting alcohol is imperative once you experience some of the long-term effects such as problems with memory and concentration, insomnia, or increased tension and conflict in relationships. As the most frequently used addictive substance in America, the National Council on Alcoholism and Drug Dependence (NCADD) has shown that alcohol hinders neurotransmitter transmission, movement, and absorption once the body has become habituated to it. When alcohol enters the brain, it causes an increase in levels of dopamine and GABA (gamma-aminobutyric acid). Both are chemical messengers produced by the brain that affect us physically and emotionally. Alcohol disrupts normal levels of these neurotransmitters, and the more the brain becomes accustomed to this interference, the more it relies on alcohol to keep these levels stable. After a person becomes dependent on alcohol, dopamine and GABA activity is altered, leading to uncomfortable and even dangerous withdrawal symptoms when they try to stop drinking.

Alcohol is quickly absorbed into the bloodstream, and its effects manifest in about 40 to 60 minutes after consumption, depending on the drink's strength. Hard liquor contains a whopping 45% alcohol, beer contains around 5% alcohol, and wine has about 15%.

Besides the havoc that binge drinking can wreak on an individual's life, chronic alcohol abuse is the leading cause of liver cancer. This disease claims the lives of thousands of people a year, causing an average of 12 fatalities per 100,000 people annually. The liver is responsible for metabolizing alcohol, and it takes 60 minutes or more to metabolize a glass of beer. Higher concentrations and over-indulgence escalate the blood-alcohol level, taking an increasingly high toll on the liver. The liver will eventually deteriorate because it's the primary filter for the toxins found in the alcohol. As residual fatty acids collect over time, the liver becomes depleted and ultimately fails to function. This condition, in turn, can give rise to alcoholic hepatitis followed by the buildup of fibrosis and scarring of the liver itself. The alarming rate at which liver disease manifests as liver cancer is another serious adverse effect.

No amount of alcohol consumption is entirely safe and when it comes to alcohol addiction, that always starts with one "quick drink" until the imbiber loses count. Recent empirical evidence collected at the University of Washington has shown that even a small amount of alcohol in the bloodstream is unsafe. "The idea that one or two drinks are safe for health is a myth," stated Dr. Emmanuela Gakidou, a senior author and professor at the University of Washington. The "one drink per day is okay" rule has been investigated, and it's been proven that even one drink is detrimental to the body and puts an individual at a higher risk of premature mortality.

In a society where drinking alcohol is associated with celebrations and good times, the growing number of alcohol addicts shouldn't be a surprise. Socioeconomic factors, genetics, gender, age, and even race play a vital role in an individual's exposure to and dependence upon alcohol, but blaming it on aspects outside of our control doesn't seem fair. Psychological factors and behavioral patterns are somewhat under our control and strongly influence our relationship with alcohol. Recent research deemed alcoholism a "disease" that manipulates the brain's neurochemistry. These changes in the brain hinder an individual's ability to control their actions. The effects of the disease, however, vary from person to person.

Since indulgence plays a significant role in many social interactions, drinking was earlier looked upon as something "healthy" if done in moderation. With modern science countering that school of thought through testimonies and evidence, it's safe to state that the supposed benefits fail to outnumber the risks attached to consumption. It's this knowledge that led to the inception of the idea that recovery from alcoholism is not only good but necessary.

If you've become accustomed to drinking and enjoy it, withdrawal may seem quite challenging. However, the road to recovery is never out of reach, and if you stay true to your commitment to stop drinking, you're halfway there. The path to sobriety is long, but you can stay on track with the right mindset and dedication.

Let's begin by acknowledging that no one picked up a glass of wine with the idea of risking their life by developing a fatal condition. Rehabilitation from alcohol is an intense process that requires maximum dedication. As a wise man once said, "Everything begins with a thought, and thoughts are turned into plans, and plans are turned into actions."

Please note that I'm not a doctor, a therapist, or a licensed professional. This book doesn't intend to replace the help of a medical professional. This book is meant to aid you on your recovery journey, and I encourage you to seek advice from your doctor or mental health care provider.

With that being said, you can embark on the road to recovery right here, right now, by deciding this is what you want to do. It's time to take your power back. It's time to take your life back and be the person you always wished to be. It's time to love yourself again. So, without any further ado, let's begin.

Chapter 1 - Alcohol in Our Culture

"First you take a drink, then the drink takes a drink, then the drink takes you."
– F. Scott Fitzgerald

Alcohol has long been regarded as a sweet relief throughout human history. The fermented beverage originated from fruit, vegetables, and even honey in the Neolithic era, evolving into what we now know as vodka, whiskey, brandy, vermouth, cognac, beer, and more. Chemically known as "ethyl" alcohol or ethanol, it's been prepared and consumed by humans for at least 7,000 years of human history. From the southeast of Asia to ancient Egypt, alcohol predates most of recorded history, with China considered to be its area of origin. The Babylonians worshiped a wine goddess in 2,700 B.C., while the Greeks shunned alcohol consumption in their earliest literature. The fact remains that alcohol has been a part of popular culture all across the globe since time immemorial.

Indigenous peoples of the Americas developed grain-based alcohol in the form of "chicha," a beverage prepared from fermented corn, grapes, and apples. Alcohol served as a medicinal additive in the 1600s and, in the 18th century, it was termed "spirits" in acknowledgment of its alchemic properties.

The mid 18th century witnessed a reform in the consumption of alcohol. What was once used as an additive to medication was now favored as an after-hours beverage when the British Parliament encouraged the use of grain to produce distilled spirits. This led to a skyrocketing demand for gin, with its consumption peaking at 18 million gallons. Great Britain became a country that encouraged drinking.

In the early 19th century, alcohol was finally recognized as an unhealthy drink, and the drinking of it needed to be discouraged. Hence, the emergence of the Temperance Movement. Later on, this movement evolved into zero tolerance toward alcohol, which was heartily rejected in America. It wasn't until 1920 that the US took legal action to ban the trade of alcohol on an international scale, but even that had little effect. The ban—called Prohibition—didn't stop people from making, buying, selling, or drinking alcohol and gave rise to the illegal alcohol trade in the 1930s. Prohibition in America ended in 1933.

Today, approximately 15 million Americans are regarded as alcoholics.

Reflection, Imitation, Social Experiences

In a society that supports alcohol use, social influence is where it all begins. Studies reveal the correlation between alcoholism and its "partners in crime," i.e., the social situations that encourage drinking. Having a drink with friends plays a significant role in the spread of alcoholism. The influence of people over their peers shows that the desire to be socially accepted can lead to alcoholism (Dallas et al., 2014; Larsen, Engels, Granic, & Overbeek, 2009; Larsen, Engels, Souren, Granic, & Overbeek, 2010). In addition, these studies revealed that the number of drinks per person increases as the number of people in a group of friends increases. However, a predisposition to alcoholism is the main culprit. Recent findings suggest an individual's likelihood of indulgence is more significant when they've already adapted to social situations that involve liberal drinking of alcohol. In simpler words, individuals are more likely to experience social bonding through drinking with others if they've been introduced to this idea growing up. (Creswell et al., 2012).

Imitating others by drinking alcohol is an attempt to promote bonding among people at social events that have drinking as a customary practice. Looking at this another way, it's somewhat awkward not to eat when everyone around you is eating, and it's the same with drinking alcohol. From a scientific point of view, eating may be a form of imitation, but drinking is associated more with people seeking validation among their peers. Social acceptance is what the "people pleaser" seeks, and drinking makes this seem more accessible.

Alcohol Use Around Us

From an accompaniment to Mediterranean cuisine to "happy hour," alcohol has become a staple in just about every culture. Its use is becoming more widespread, driven by misconceptions that thrive in our collective societies. As we've seen, alcohol was once widely considered as something healthy. "A glass of wine a day keeps the doctor away" was the excuse that indulgers would use since there's evidence that certain types of alcohol (red wine, primarily) help prevent heart disease. However, this claim was rejected by a global study published in *The Lancet* that analyzed the effects of alcohol on consumers in 195 countries over 16 years. The results concluded that the effects of alcohol consumption greatly outweigh the benefits. So-called "moderate drinking" has many negative repercussions, with an enhanced risk of cancer being among them.

"The safest amount of alcohol is none," was the verdict of this research. The study analyzed a wide range of adverse effects related directly to alcohol consumption, from drunken driving incidents to self-harm and more. What was severely disturbing was the big reveal that almost 10% of early deaths in people in the 15-to-49 age group were due to alcohol consumption.

The Alcohol Illusion

Let's admit it. Alcohol doesn't taste good, it doesn't benefit you in any way, and it costs a lot too. So why is it that we still tend to associate alcohol with "good times?" The inclination toward indulgence begins relatively early, and while we all shun the idea of early drinking, it's encouraged when we become adults. The damage it creates is the same, whether the drinker is a teenager or an adult, so the double standard isn't only ironic but illogical.

The belief that alcohol enhances the pleasure of other activities is nothing more than an illusion. The idea that drinking alcohol makes you appear more sophisticated and allows you to relax more is a myth. A drink of straight alcohol is anything but fun, and mixing the venom with sweeter nectars only masks the awfulness. If you're drinking more than twice a week, you're already on the addiction spectrum.

If you try to reduce your consumption, you'll feel the withdrawal effects—which often leads you to have just "one more drink," which temporarily relieves your distress. You tell yourself that was the "last," but this is where the never-ending circle of defeat begins. Just a glass will no longer satisfy you. Before you know it, you've been sucked deep into the vicious cycle of alcoholism, disease, broken relationships, career loss, and a bad reputation.

When you recognize you need more alcohol than you used to, you have a problem. This is the first and most important step. Admitting there's a problem is the hardest part for most alcoholics, but once you reach that milestone, you're already on the path to recovery.

Everyone You Know Drinks Alcohol, So How Come it's Just You Who Has a Problem?

Putting yourself under the microscope and doing "analysis to paralysis" is convenient for those in denial. You try to figure out why everyone else doesn't seem to have a problem with drinking, and you do, but you need to understand that "everyone else" isn't your concern. You're responsible for your body and your health, not theirs. In other words, you need to "mind your own business." Comparing our bad habits to those of others is a flawed approach to begin with. There's no competition here, so why do you need to compare your experiences with those of others?

Different bodies have different metabolism rates, so the effects of alcohol differ from person to person. However, it's an addictive substance no matter who the person is. Statistics prove the repercussions of alcohol abuse don't discriminate against age, race, or gender. Denial isn't the way to go.

Notice if you have any of these symptoms of alcohol addiction:

- You're losing count of the number of shots you're gulping down.
- You feel sick more often after drinking.
- You're no longer as sensitive to the effects of alcohol, and it fails to give you a buzz.
- The craving is getting out of hand.
- Life is less fun.
- You're becoming more aggressive.
- You need to drink to get through the day.
- You're becoming reckless.
- You keep getting sick.
- Other areas of your life are starting to suffer.

From a scientific point of view, research has shown that the body's metabolism determines the effects of alcohol. The metabolism of alcohol, in turn, is greatly influenced by genetic factors, environmental factors, and the amount of alcohol consumed. In a nutshell, alcoholism is influenced by the factors discussed earlier in the chapter—the predisposition to drinking alcohol, social imitation, and life experiences.

What Is Alcoholism?

The biochemistry of ethyl alcohol in the body is a complex science. Alcohol was the seventh leading cause of death globally in 2016, which prompted an updated analysis of its molecular biology by *The Lancet* (1873a). Metabolized predominantly by the liver, the effects of alcohol initially manifest in the central nervous system—hence its impact on social behavior. However, its delayed effects are even more severe.

Alcohol is metabolized by several pathways. The two most significant processes involve two enzymes— dehydrogenase (ADH) and aldehyde dehydrogenase (ALDH)—which aid in breaking down ethanol. ADH converts alcohol to acetaldehyde, a highly toxic substance that's been identified as a carcinogen. Later in the process, acetaldehyde is metabolized into acetate, which, in turn, is broken down into water and carbon dioxide. You might believe that since the end products of alcohol metabolism are just water and carbon dioxide, it would be harmless, but there's a lot more to it than that. The toxicity involved in the process takes a toll on the liver. Not just that, alcohol also damages the pancreas, the brain, the heart, and the central nervous system. As mentioned previously, alcohol is implicated in liver cancer.

What Does It Mean to Get Drunk? What Does It Mean to Have a Hangover?

It takes the liver from one to two hours to metabolize alcohol into its constituent compounds. When the number of drinks exceeds the liver's efficiency, we witness the "drunken" state taking effect. A hangover, which typically occurs after a night of excessive alcohol consumption, is primarily caused by dehydration and electrolyte imbalances that lead to headache, nausea, stomach cramps, light sensitivity, dizziness, poor sleep, inflammation, and vomiting.

Legally, being "drunk" occurs when the blood alcohol content (BOC) is 0.08 or higher, with anything close to 0.40 usually being fatal. The drunken state may be visible in an individual's coordination, balance, speech, and reflexes. An excessively high blood-alcohol level will hinder an individual's ability to see, stay awake, and focus when needed. Drinking large amounts of alcohol in a short period of time will worsen the effects and can lead to alcohol poisoning, coma, and even death.

What Is an Alcoholic?

The word "alcoholic" may bring to mind the picture of a sad, slightly overweight, blue-collar male with a bottle of beer who's facing a mid-life crisis. However, it isn't always easy to identify an alcoholic. Alcoholism can affect people from all walks of life—from teenagers to the elderly, rich or poor. Celebrities with great looks and prosperous careers like Anna Nicole Smith and John Barrymore lost their lives to alcoholism, so appearances can indeed be deceiving.

The very first tell-tale signs of an alcoholic include the following red flags:

- Appearing to be in a state of intoxication most of the time.
- No constraints on drinking, be it at work or after hours.
- The urge to drink increases, and so does the amount or strength of the liquor.

- A tired appearance and a cranky attitude.
- Inefficiency.
- A lack of interest in ordinary life.
- Being sad and depressed most of the time.
- Dishonest and secretive.

An individual displaying some of these signs may be an alcoholic. Still, since society has stigmatized the word as something humiliating, we might refrain from terming an individual with a drinking problem an alcoholic to spare the sufferer shame and even scandal. Because of the widespread availability of alcohol at just about any social event and its acceptance by our society, it seems unfair to blame alcoholism on its victims.

Some schools of thought opt for the "tough love" approach of shaming the alcoholic in an effort to help the individual abstain from drinking, but this method rarely works. A guilt-ridden intoxicated person is likely to indulge even more in the habit, and in extreme cases, they may even contemplate suicide. The burden of being an "alcoholic" is heavy, and blaming the sufferer isn't helpful. A proactive approach is needed, with counseling being the primary step.

Alcohol Damage

Addiction takes varying lengths of time to become established depending on the individual, but what remains consistent is the tolerance to alcohol that builds up, which occurs in anyone who drinks regularly. A particular individual may be more susceptible to the damaging effects of alcohol, while another might be less so. Over time, regular alcohol consumption causes an imbalance in gamma-aminobutyric acid (GABA), a neurotransmitter responsible for controlling impulsivity. Not only that, alcoholism disrupts the balance of glutamate, another neurotransmitter that's responsible for sending signals to other types of cells in the body.

Dopamine is also a neurotransmitter, and when dopamine levels in the brain increase, we experience pleasure. Over time, the brain becomes addicted to the release of dopamine, which is one of the roots of addiction. The body requires more and more dopamine release to experience the euphoria of pleasure.

If a person consumes large amounts of alcohol regularly, their tolerance can increase, and the body requires more alcohol to achieve the desired effect. This will, lead to the development of life-threatening diseases like cancer of the breast, mouth, esophagus, voice box, colon, rectum, and throat. Other conditions may include high blood pressure, liver disease, chronic digestive issues, and more.

The Cost of Drinking

The Centers for Disease Control and Prevention (CDC) estimate that alcoholism costs the US economy $249 billion each year. This breaks down to $28 billion in healthcare costs, $179 billion in loss of workplace productivity, $25 billion in alcohol-related criminal justice cases, and $13 billion in accidents and collisions.

On a smaller scale, an individual will pay around $10 per drink in a bar or dining establishment, depending on the brand of alcohol and how upscale the venue where it's being purchased. Seldom does an individual at a bar or restaurant stop at a single drink. According to CDC stats, a male consumer typically drinks four to 14 drinks per week, and an average female will consume four to seven alcoholic beverages per week. The cost of alcoholism doesn't end there. Broken relationships, DUI tickets, healthcare expenses, job loss, and lost opportunities make alcoholism one of the most costly bad habits.

In total, alcohol-related conditions and illness are estimated to cost NHS England about £3.5 billion annually, so it's not just a serious problem in the USA. Alcoholism is a global issue, and its real-time costs manifest in healthcare, family life, efficiency on the job, and other aspects. These can't be accurately measured, so it's impossible to put a dollar amount on its effects in these areas. All the more disturbing is that an alarming percentage of alcohol use disorder (AUD) sufferers eventually resort to drug abuse, making alcohol abuse directly related to drug abuse. By digging deeper into all the mishaps and losses associated with drugs, you might be able to comprehend to some extent the amount of damage alcohol causes, economically and otherwise.

Chapter 2 - Understanding Your Habits and Needs

"The initial journey towards sobriety is a delicate balance between insight into one's desire for escape and abstinence from one's addiction." — Debra L. Kaplan

The Basics of Habits

Abraham Maslow, an American psychiatrist, defined psychotherapy as having the element of "self" as its cornerstone. With the advent of the modern-day "self-actualization" theme, Millennials and their counterparts in Gen Z and Gen X have perverted this theory into an excuse for a night out binge drinking. This is how alcoholic habits begin.

Bad habits originate from four basic steps: the cue, the craving, the response, and the reward. With drinking, the cue is initiated when you intentionally set out to drink. With something as available and addictive as alcohol, the pattern can set in quite easily, and before you know it, the craving phase begins. The response is when you satisfy those cravings, and the reward is the feeling of false contentment you get when you reach a state of intoxication. A *New York Times* bestseller, *The Atomic Habit*, defined life as the sum of our habits. If drinking has become a habit, what does that mean for your life? Now *there's* some food for thought.

Your Most Fundamental Needs

Looking at Maslow"s Hierarchy of Needs, we know that alcohol doesn't fit into the pyramid anywhere at all, so it's not a "need" to begin with. The top of the pyramid is "self-actualization," which encourages innovation, creativity, growth, and abundance—none of which alcohol facilitates. To reach the top of the hierarchy, the lower-down needs must be met. Physical needs such as food, shelter, sleep, and clothing are the first step, followed by the second tier in the hierarchy, safety needs. Safety needs doesn't just refer to protection from robbers and losses. They also have to do with emotional stability, well-being, and financial security—all things that alcohol can rob you of.

The third tier is the need to be loved and belong. Family bonds and social activities occupy this slot. Alcohol is the main culprit in ruining family bonds and can even bring out aggression in an individual. Sharing your drinking hobby at a bar with a friend might fulfill the needs of being loved and belonging for those few moments, but this isn't a healthy or sustainable means for getting those.

The fourth step in the pyramid is "esteem needs." This refers to an individual's need for self-respect, acknowledgment, and appreciation for their achievements and existence. Alcohol significantly hinders this aspect of one's life. Being an alcoholic robs you of your self-respect and, eventually, your social status as well. It undermines your potential and blocks you from achieving your goals.

Your Needs as an Alcohol Drinker

Alcoholism is another term for alcohol abuse. Once we acknowledge we're an alcoholic, we can get on the path to recovery. This is where positive changes begin, but the alcoholic must first analyze their needs as an individual with AUD. Those needs should revolve around abstaining from alcohol.

Let's discuss the possible methods an alcoholic might use to move into abstinence:

- The DIY approach: Before you resort to rehab, you can always begin at home. Remove all alcohol from your home. If it's not easily in reach, you're more likely to control your drinking behavior.

- Address your demons: There could be underlying problems in your surroundings that trigger you into grabbing a drink. Are you in a toxic relationship? Does your job play a role in stressing you out to the point where you often feel you need a drink? Are you suffering from depression, trauma, or other mental illness? Compromised mental health can play a significant role in alcoholism.

- Stay proactive: Keeping numbers of supportive people or organizations saved in your phone is a crucial step. Free information about quitting drinking is available on the internet and in e-books that will help you understand alcoholism.

- Notice your patterns. A pattern refers to a state of mind that leads an individual into a specific behavior. Study your patterns. If you notice a pattern, it will be easier for you to remove what triggers you into grabbing a drink. Moreover, a counselor can help you figure out a plan that will prevent you from falling back into an unhealthy pattern. In cases that require deeper inner work, cognitive behavioral therapy can help individuals regain their balance.

- Support: It's always wise to brief your immediate family about an addiction problem. Professional programs can help with recovery by offering group therapy, activity therapy, and more.

Understanding Why You Drink

As mentioned earlier, the common reasons why people drink include social acceptance, temporarily escaping stress, enhancing pleasure, and, in some folks, bringing out the daredevil in them. A study conducted at PMC Labs found that the two primary causes of heavy drinking are negative reinforcement and positive reinforcement. The former implies that an individual drinks as a coping mechanism to avoid feelings of hopelessness, sadness, and depression. The latter has to do with "letting loose" and being more sociable. Cahalan et al. (1969) described the two different groups of drinkers in more detail, indicating that social reasons for drinking were associated more with lighter drinkers while abusive drinking had more to do with individuals trying to cope with problems. Nonetheless, the findings support the premise that social drinking can still lead to alcoholism.

This study found increased indulgence in the negative-reinforcement group when they were faced with situations that exacerbated their stress, whereas the positive-reinforcement group drank more when socializing more. The two groups were further broken down into gender, ethnicity, and age. The study revealed that males were better able to cope with stress without overdrinking than were women. Yet, men are more likely to be alcoholics than women. The study had some conflicting results. The final conclusion was that any individual with a craving for alcohol will give in to the urge now and then, regardless of whether their motive is driven by negative or positive reinforcement.

Alcohol, in its essence, is a depressant. Clinically defined as a sedative, it numbs the senses and changes an individual's emotional responses.

In light of Maslow's Hierarchy of Needs, where does that leave the AUD sufferer? What are your reasons for drinking? You may no longer have a reason because addiction has taken away your ability to choose your behavior.

Do You Have a Problem with Alcohol?

Before we begin to dissect the details of alcohol addiction, let's first address the elephant in the room: Are you a problem drinker? If so, can you admit this, or are you in denial? Studies reveal that the acceptance of being an alcohol abuser aids tremendously in an individual's recovery. However, some individuals are genuinely clueless about whether they've developed an alcohol addiction. The following questions will help you identify your status regarding alcohol use:

- Do you end up drinking more than you planned to?
- Does your usual amount of drinks work the way they used to?
- Would you rather drink than indulge in a favorite hobby or pastime?
- Have you tried to quit drinking and failed to do so?
- Do you crave alcohol?
- How much time do you spend drinking?
- Is drinking becoming a problem for the people around you?

- Have you gotten into any sort of trouble because of drinking?
- Has drinking landed you in dangerous situations like tickets for DUI or fights?
- Do you suffer withdrawal symptoms when you refrain from drinking?

Answers to these questions will help reveal your relationship with alcohol, but a deeper approach from a medical standpoint is needed. Blood tests aid in assessing whether an individual has been drinking heavily for a prolonged period. Lab work can indicate a decrease in red blood cells, which is a symptom of prolonged alcohol abuse. Testing for carbohydrate-deficient transferrin (CDT) can reveal if a person has been drinking excessive amounts of alcohol daily or has relapsed after not drinking for a while. Other tests may be needed to analyze a binge drinker's liver damage and reduced testosterone levels in men.

How Much Do You Drink?

The road to alcoholism is a confusing one. From pints to goblets, martini glasses to shots, understanding the amount of alcohol in a particular drink is a science in its own right. On top of that is the task of keeping score of how much you drink, which can be quite the ordeal. How does the layman even know how much a "unit" of alcohol is so they can track their consumption? A unit is the measure introduced in the UK in 1987 to help people track the amount of alcohol they consume. One unit equals 10 ml or 0.34 fl oz of alcohol—the amount the liver metabolizes in about an hour. In simpler words, a unit of alcohol should take approximately one hour to leave the body.

Keeping score of the amount of alcohol entering your body can help in determining whether you have alcoholism. It might sound a bit contradictory, given that we stated earlier that no amount of alcohol is safe, but keeping track of consumption is sometimes the only way for an abuser to wean themselves from their habit. Apart from that, a zero-tolerance attitude toward liquor is an unrealistic idea for most people. Keeping tabs on the number of drinks consumed seems more practical if the concept of abstinence seems impossible.

It's been recommended that men and women refrain from consuming more than 14 units of alcohol a week. It's much healthier to spread this consumption over several days in a week rather than imbibing the 14 units in one go. If a drinker can reduce their consumption from two drinks a day to one, they're well on their way to refraining from drinking at all for two or three days. This is how the body is trained into returning to normal and functioning well without the daily alcohol dose. There may be withdrawal symptoms, but with this step-down regimen, they won't be as severe.

For anyone trying to wean off of alcohol completely, be aware that becoming sober is more challenging than falling into alcoholism. But remember, when the going gets tough, the tough get going. There will be days in which you'll feel sick to the bone, and there will be times when you may relapse. Know that this is all a part of the process. To save your precious life, there's no other way but to accept the minor setbacks and keep going forward with your plan to be clean and sober.

What Does it Mean to Stop Drinking Alcohol?

This is the essence of the campaign you've begun: What does it mean if you stop drinking alcohol? Are you thinking about abstaining from just the drink, or is it a complete lifestyle you're willing to let go of to stay sober? There's a lot more than what meets the eye with alcoholism. Just as alcohol affects people differently, the reasons why an individual wants to quit alcohol vary from person to person. For some, it might be to regain the healthy appearance they once had. For others, they want to avoid the sickening hangover. Others may wish to stop drinking for spiritual or religious reasons. Individuals may even try sobriety as a weight-loss plan because alcohol can lead to obesity.

The reason you want to quit alcohol should be crystal clear in your mind because it plays a vital role in your willpower. With something as addictive and dangerous as alcohol, the decision to quit should be first discussed with a health professional. In almost every country, there are government agencies to aid you with free services and counseling all along your journey.

Quitting alcohol "cold turkey" carries serious risks for alcoholics, so a professional's supervision is required to help the individual through the acute withdrawal phase.

Withdrawal symptoms range from nausea, trembling, dizziness, sleeplessness, cold sweats, and even heart palpitations to convulsions and hallucinations. These symptoms can be severe, and being under close observation may be essential for some people. A professional may help relieve the symptoms with medication, counseling, and psychological support. Programs are designed to allocate a team of professionals to help the person through this process. Signing up with a support system in your vicinity is highly recommended to maintain your sobriety.

Recognizing You Have a Problem

Alcohol abuse can cripple your life in many ways. The list is a long one. Alcoholism can be deadly, and health complications are sometimes irreversible. With all the evidence of the harm that alcohol can cause and the help available to treat alcohol abuse, it's still a long road from disease to recovery, which calls for some in-depth analysis. Alcoholism is curable, yet the death toll doesn't seem to dwindle.

Information online explores every aspect of research but overlooks a crucial and obvious factor: denial of being an alcoholic. Alcoholics are unwilling to admit that alcoholism puts them in danger of an early death and plays a significant role in their diminishing health. Denial prevents individuals from seeking help that can lead to recovery, reduces their chances of survival, prevents them from gaining control of their lives, and sends them into a downward spiral. Denial is common in alcohol abusers—especially those who perished from the disease.

Indulgers may play the blame game quite well, and that, too, is a form of denial as is rationalizing their relationship with alcohol. Instead of falling prey to denial, you must acknowledge the problem and admit you're abusing alcohol. Being defensive about a bad habit only delays your recovery. Value your life, and recognize you have a problem. Once you accept your mistakes, you can begin your journey to recovery.

What Are Your Reasons for Considering Quitting Alcohol?

Once you've accepted that you have a problem, it's time to narrow down the options for how to address it. What are the reasons you want to quit drinking? It's usually not because your doctor or your family told you to. Why did you start drinking? What caused you to seek refuge in alcohol? Was it a catastrophic event that led you to start drinking? Was it a relationship? Is drinking a way for you to process grief and past trauma? Once you know the reasons for why you drink, you can see how alcoholism was never the answer and how it only made your problems worse.

Understanding what made you turn to alcohol will help sustain you in your efforts. In the past several decades, alcohol use amongst teenagers has increased. According to surveys conducted at the request of TeensHealth, one of the main factors that contribute to underage drinking is peer pressure. The false promise in mainstream media that drinking makes an individual "feel better" is another significant reason for the rise in alcohol use amongst teens. Another contributor is an unstable home life leading to alcohol use as a coping mechanism. The reasons for alcohol abuse amongst teens are very similar to those of adults who abuse alcohol.

Once the reason behind alcoholism is identified, it can be acknowledged. After that, the next step is to realize that sobriety has more to do with your mindset than your cravings. If you have a clear perspective on what you want for your life, you'll be successful.

Denial

As mentioned previously, "denial" is a predominant factor that sets you back from recovery. You outright deny you have a problem with alcohol, and you're unable or unwilling to admit your dependency.

The denial aspect is the most frustrating factor for those dealing with another's alcohol abuse problem. It may cause the individual's support team to become discouraged. It can even happen that the problem drinker's friends and family start to deny there's a problem. When denial is too overpowering, the only way out is for the alcoholic to eventually admit they have a problem rather than blaming their habit on the people around them, their life situation, or "fate." Common excuses of deniers include, "He/She ruined my life," "He/She dumped me," "I have no other way out but to drink," or "Alcohol is the only way I can numb the pain." These excuses are usually accompanied by an arrogant attitude. A problem drinker will deny their breath smells of alcohol or give a weak excuse for drinking: "I purchased the bottle of wine for guests coming over," or "I stopped by at the pub for a meeting." The more you confront them, the more defensive they get. At times, it's just the "I'll do as I please" refrain and, at other times, it's the "Just one drink" song-and-dance. Confrontation is the hardest part of the process. An alcoholic is rarely ready to admit they have a problem when confronted. At times, even the parents and friends will be lied to and given excuses.

Sometimes, the sufferer will agree with you that they need to stop, although they have no intention of doing this. They'll say, "You're right. From today onwards,

I'm not touching a drop." As soon as you're out of sight, they're off in search of a drink. Denial may even involve comparing themselves to someone else with explanations like, "George has been drinking all his life, he's older than I am, and he's doing pretty good."

Denial has many faces, but the longer abusers downplay their addiction, the greater the risk of ill health or death.

You Aren't Alone

Instead of beating around the bush and gambling with your life, it's essential to confront your addiction, even if it may seem excessive to admit you're an alcoholic. The CDC estimates 4.5% of men and 2.5% of women suffer from alcoholism, so it's certainly not just you who has a problem—nor is it your fault. One in every three households in the US has someone in their extended social circle who suffers from alcohol abuse. The fact that the disease is still stigmatized has significantly hindered awareness of it on a mass scale.

Drinking a can of beer is considered a harmless social

act, yet alcoholism carries a stigma. Individuals with AUD are under pressure to keep their addiction a secret, which only fuels denial. Secrets ruin lives. It's enough that you suffer from alcoholism. You don't need to go through it alone. Know that there's always help if only you reach out. If you have a judgmental family, try opening up to a friend. Contact a professional if friends aren't understanding—or are alcohol abusers themselves. Don't feel embarrassed to suffer from a condition that's plagued humanity for centuries.

On a more objective note, alcoholism rarely occurs in just one family member. Drug addiction and alcoholism are often considered "family illnesses." This means addiction can be contagious—just like social drinking—even though it's not viral. Put simply, alcoholism is more likely if a close family member is an alcoholic. Frequently, family will try to intervene to help an alcoholic family member, but since the disease is complex, they're often not successful. If you're suffering from alcohol abuse, you have a greater chance of having someone around you who's walked the same path. Former sufferers can help an alcoholic better since they know what it's like.

Hitting Rock Bottom

Alcohol use disorder is a health concern on a global scale. Whether it's viewed as a social evil or just a bad habit, the fact remains that the disorder has wreaked havoc on countless lives. Many individuals suffering from AUD fail to address the problem effectively. Research has revealed that "hitting rock bottom" is a crucial factor in motivating an individual to stop drinking and save their life. From the indulger's perspective, hitting rock bottom is when they finally acknowledge they need help with their AUD.

What constitutes rock bottom is different for each individual. For some, it might be the near-death experience of alcohol poisoning. For others, it may be that their spouse walked out on them because of their AUD. Hitting rock bottom has been termed the tipping point that compels individuals to seek treatment (Cunningham et al., 1994). However, the phenomenon of "rock bottom" has never been defined in terms of specific signs and symptoms, so the definition remains subjective.

As dangerous as hitting rock bottom may sound, it's helped individuals climb back up to sobriety. The experience has been primarily defined as the alcoholic awakening to the realization that one more drink or one more binge may be their last. They may see their life flashing before their eyes and understand that it's now or never. It's at this point that they get serious about sobriety.

Moderation: One Drink at a Time

As mentioned earlier, alcohol addiction comes with a price. Even when you decide to get rid of the demon, it continues to haunt you with a vengeance. Withdrawal symptoms can leave a person debilitated, and going cold turkey makes the symptoms even worse. Heart palpitations, sleeplessness, lack of appetite, cold sweats, a constant state of anxiety, convulsions, and shivering are a few of the symptoms an alcoholic may face in their quest for sobriety.

Consuming alcohol puts you at risk of heart disease,

several types of cancer, cirrhosis, a compromised quality of life, and plenty of DUI tickets. On the other hand, stopping drinking can set you up for debilitating withdrawal symptoms. So, where does that leave you? Seeking to become sober may at times have you feeling torn between saving your life or giving up on it altogether. Nonetheless, there's a way out. The sweet spot in the quest for sobriety is called "moderation."

The moderation approach is the more practical way to achieve sobriety. Just as stopping certain medications abruptly has its drawbacks, the same is true of alcohol. Moderation allows you to gradually wean off alcohol to allow your body to slowly adjust to what it's become dependent on.

For an alcoholic, drinking alcohol even occasionally is highly discouraged. However, an occasional drink is sometimes necessary for the sake of their well-being. While the recommended moderate alcohol intake is limited to two drinks or fewer a day for men and one drink or fewer a day for women, an addict may need more or less of the recommended moderate amount depending on their body and addiction scenario.

Sobriety

Commonly described as turning away from alcoholism, "sobriety" is somewhat misunderstood. Although the term refers to complete abstinence from alcohol, it has to do with more than just alcohol. Sobriety is, in fact, a change of lifestyle. The most effective measures along the path to sobriety often include changing your circle of friends and your regular hangouts. It's a thorough reforming of your life and requires total commitment.

Sobriety is often regarded as freedom from drug abuse, alcohol, or other substances. In a more profound sense, sobriety is an ongoing process of recovery. The approach to sobriety addresses the root cause of the substance abuse, how it took control over the individual's life, and how they can get back on track. Be it the addiction itself, a hidden psychological condition that led to it, or a coping mechanism to escape the stresses of life, sobriety addresses all of these. It focuses on freeing the individual from everything related to their bad habit, from their past and into their future. The process may even involve mental health therapy and spiritual healing along with medical detox.

The benefits of sobriety range from a general sense of well-being to improved relationships. A few of the benefits of being sober include:

- Improved memory (no brain fog and better critical thinking and decision-making skills)
- Healthier skin
- Improved overall appearance
- Improved sleep
- Decreased risk of cancer
- Better weight management
- Healthier eating habits
- Improved testosterone levels
- Slower aging
- Decreased inflammation

While sobriety allows your internal organs to recover from alcohol-induced damage and, hence, improve your physical health, it will also allow you to see how drinking was damaging your relationships with the people around you. Emotional stability is one of the most significant benefits sobriety provides to the addict. Much like how drinking primarily affects the central nervous system—causing anxiety, tremors, and other afflictions—abstinence initiates the repair of the nervous system to health within the first few days.

Chapter 3 – First Steps to Freedom

"You don't have to see the whole staircase. Just take the first step." – Martin Luther King

Professional Help and Support

Alcoholism is the gateway to a myriad of problems. The irony is, many of the initial symptoms are often brushed under the rug. Even though alcoholism is among the most significant public health concerns in the United States, the issue still fails to receive adequate attention.

Many individuals find it hard to control their drinking behavior at some point in their lives. In the US, nearly 15 million people have been diagnosed with AUD, with one in 10 children living with a parent with AUD. Treatment of AUD does, in fact, work wonders. Regardless of how severe the problem, there's always hope. A combination of mental health support and medical treatment can free an individual from the fatal grasp of AUD.

An individual should immediately seek professional help if they experience any of the following symptoms:

- Memory problems
- Cold sweats
- Heart palpitations
- Yellowing of the skin and eyes
- Swelling in the legs
- Bruising easily
- Vomiting blood
- Dark urine and tarry looking feces
- A swollen abdomen

The above symptoms need immediate medical intervention, as they may indicate advanced alcoholism. However, a proactive approach is a much better way to avoid the emergency room. Symptoms of alcoholism that signal the need for professional help and support include depression, restlessness, anxiety, nausea, sweating, insomnia, and irritability.

Individuals on the milder spectrum of the disease should reach out to support groups that can help in the initial stages of AUD. Help is readily available online, which also allows you to remain anonymous if you wish. There are verified agencies like the Substance Abuse and Mental Help Services Administration, BetterHelp, and the National Institute on Alcohol Abuse and Alcoholism. You can start the process with a phone call or by filling out an online form. Before you know it, you're in a support group where you can begin to share your concerns. Communication is vital, so don't be afraid to let it all out.

Support groups allow individuals to talk to people who are or have been in their shoes and know what it feels like to suffer from alcoholism. Group chats and professional intervention may aid sufferers in many ways. Counseling is a crucial step on the road to recovery.

Expectations

When it comes to sobriety, expectations are often far from reality. This book doesn't provide an overnight fix to something as debilitating as alcohol addiction. It is, however, a guide for embarking on that journey and tackling the problem one step at a time. As mentioned earlier, the liver takes about an hour to metabolize one unit of alcohol. The more you drink, the longer it takes for the liver to flush the alcohol from the body, let alone the toxins it contains that damage the liver and other organs. Breaking the habit takes a lot more conviction than developing it.

To break the cycle, the basic 20-day rule applies. It's said that it takes 20 days, on average, to break a habit. With alcoholism, an individual can try the 20-day rule to see where they stand. Don't go easy on yourself during that period. Abstinence can assist in decreasing tolerance to alcohol, making drinking in moderation possible. If you don't indulge your urge for those 20 days, try for 40 days. If nothing else, your body could use the break.

Withdrawal symptoms begin almost immediately, so expect the first week to be tough. You may experience the following symptoms in those weeks:

- Palpitations
- Breathlessness
- Dizziness
- Sleeplessness
- Nausea
- Diminished appetite
- Paranoia

Once you overcome these obstacles, you'll know you're capable of surviving the ride ahead. Sometimes, symptoms are severe, and you may even need to be hospitalized. Medications like neuroleptics and benzodiazepines may be required along with a diet plan. A bleak side-effect of sobriety is the risk of experiencing seizures, but proper medication can minimize the chances of these happening. Withdrawal symptoms and the accompanying treatment may seem to be a huge turnoff, but the initial difficult stages of recovery are necessary for getting your life back. Keep an open mind and shift your focus to the new "you" waiting on the other end of the process.

Mindset

For most people, becoming sober doesn't work on the first attempt. The road to sobriety is a rollercoaster ride, and there will be times when you'll feel discouraged about ever getting sober. Sobriety itself is a hard road, and there will likely be episodes of relapse, binge drinking, and a return of sobriety. The key to success is your willpower and your perseverance. The right mindset is what will pull you through.

Understand that it's your life at stake. You didn't come this far to die an addict. Think about who you aspired to become when you were younger and what alcohol turned you into. You could have achieved better things had you not fallen for something as insignificant as a bad-tasting beverage in a glass. For your future and the sake of your loved ones, you have to reboot your life and start anew each time you relapse. Brighter days are awaiting you, so you must regain your health.

Adapting a "growth mindset" has helped individuals move forward following setbacks. A growth mindset is a practical approach to conquering your addiction. It encourages the belief that you'll be successful in your efforts regardless of how many times you've failed. Believing you're in complete control of your abilities can help you improve and progress. This is the true key to success. With the right attitude, individuals will strengthen their willpower and pull themselves through.

With such a tough adversary as alcoholism, it's okay if you relapse. All you need to do is get back up and continue on the road to sobriety. Don't give up until you get there—and you will. Persistence, effort, and hard work are critical, but they aren't as important as believing you're in control of your destiny.

Preparation

Addiction isn't one of those things in life that you

should rely on luck to help you overcome. Quitting an active addiction takes a strong will, focus, and preplanning for you to be successful. This doesn't even take into consideration the amount of effort you need to stay in recovery or maintain sobriety.

As any good self-help book or coach will tell you, success comes from proper planning and preparation. While it may seem that people who successfully achieve their goals do this through luck or that one single break, we often only see the tip of the iceberg of the work that went into that specific achievement. The same is true for anyone who's attempting to break free of the chains of addiction. It's easy to be overwhelmed by the idea of getting sober. There are so many things to consider and actions to take that you might feel paralyzed.

The most significant step in preparing yourself for the journey ahead is creating an action plan and committing to it. That commitment comes in two parts. The first part is committing to this process by stepping across the starting line and quitting drinking on day one. The second part is an ongoing commitment to continuously propel yourself toward your goals and move one step further away from your alcohol use each day. Believe you can do it, and you're halfway there!

The recommended action plan for alcohol recovery has four aspects: humility, motivation, perseverance in effort, and the restoration of love and purpose to your life. As the names of these four aspects suggest, the action plan has everything to do with your mental health. Let's get into the details of the action plan.

Set Short-term and Long-term Goals

Your plan has to have a time frame. We can get so caught up in the process of preparing to stop drinking that we never step over that starting line to do it. Procrastination can be a big issue when facing something that might cause you some discomfort. This is why its so important to set a specific time frame for beginning your journey and meeting your goals.

Use the following three questions to form a framework for continued action:

1.   What activities do I need to do to achieve my goal, and in what time frame?
2.   What resources do I need?
3.   Who can help me achieve my goal?

Take It One Step at a Time

Quitting alcoholism is tough, so setting out a five-year plan when you first start is illogical and farfetched. Keep it simple, and start small. Reward yourself for each step you accomplish, and reflect on your journey. Be proud of yourself for even going a day without alcohol. If you gave in to the urge, think about why you did that. There's always a reason behind the trigger. Dissect the basis and troubleshoot the problem.

Record Your Progress

Alcohol use disorder isn't just about how much you drink but also how often, so you want to record both. If you relapse, record that too. As you progress along the road to recovery, you'll have something to reflect on and become aware of the powerful effects of abstinence. You'll find that you're relapsing less than you were a couple of months ago.

No matter how lousy you may feel at times, don't let the sick days inhabit your mind. Instead, focus on who you'll be a year from now. In the worst moments, tell yourself, "This too shall pass," and believe in it.

Transitioning to sobriety is a slow and steady process with many hurdles. Use a calendar to highlight days in which you were successful. The visual markers will motivate you more than you imagine.

Find Your Support Team

We live in a world where people are constantly judged. You don't need to add to your anxiety by telling everyone about your situation. Tell your close family and friends that you're trying to stop drinking alcohol and explain why. This way, you can share your successes with them, and they'll understand why you've started declining drinks or trips to the bar. Frequently reminding yourself and the people close to you why you want to stop drinking can help keep you on track and may even encourage someone else to give up or cut down along with you.

If you prefer to keep your journey private and need moral support at any point in time, go online and sign up with a support group that keeps your identity anonymous. You can easily find a buddy who knows what you're going through and interact with them about your issues. Communication helps a lot when the person you're talking to knows what it's like.

Stay Dedicated

Recovery is all about motivation, so the reason that steered you toward sobriety should be one that you can easily find strength in. Recall this reason each time you feel like having a drink. Reflect on who you were before you started drinking or who you can be once you stop. Persevere, and keep moving forward.

Manage Triggers and Cravings

There are three primary facts about cravings that you need to bring to mind each time you have a craving: cravings are time-limited, cravings don't have to be satisfied, and ignoring a craving won't harm you—in fact, quite the contrary. An effective way to deal with a craving is to divert your attention as soon as you feel it. Take a little walk and distance yourself from the situation or people around you.

Abstaining from alcohol might seem like the best route to sobriety, but this may have some dire consequences. It may force you to avoid pubs altogether or exit social events where drinking is the norm. Individuals with a strong addiction might even avoid food that includes a "dash of alcohol." Regardless of how harsh it may seem to your friends and acquaintances, abstinence must take priority because that's what will save your life. You can always politely refuse invitations from people, and if you know them well enough, you can let them know you're trying to get sober.

Replace Old Habits with New Ones

An action plan like this will get you started on the road to recovery, but achieving the ultimate goal of total sobriety doesn't happen quickly. The action plan lays the groundwork for you to get started. Regardless of how insignificant your effort might seem compared to your addiction, the most important thing is to start. The essence of sobriety comes down to changing your daily habits. Replacing drinking with healthier habits is how you jump-start your recovery.

Alcohol addiction isn't an isolated behavior. It's always part of an unhealthy lifestyle. An unhealthy lifestyle isn't just about what you eat and drink. It includes unhealthy relationships, stress, and other types of trouble. If drinking is the compensating mechanism in dealing with a stressful relationship, job, or situation, you need to find another way to address this. We're certainly not suggesting that you abandon friends and family because they stress you out. The key is finding a way to reduce that stress.

Focus on everything that alcohol is preventing you from doing and dedicate yourself to the tasks you've long put off. Devote your time to work, family, and your well-being. Volunteering for community work is very rewarding, and you might meet people going through the same transformation that you are, at least mentally. Love and meaningful work are the greatest blessings of life, so make sure you double-dip on those two aspects.

To replace your usual "Happy Hour," try catching some coffee with a friend. You'll find more coffee drinkers than alcohol indulgers just about anywhere. Spending happy hour with friends and family at home is an even better idea. If this doesn't sound like a good vibe for you, you can always just say no to alcohol, even at a pub with friends. You can have a non-alcoholic beer, if you enjoy the taste of beer, or a club soda. You can make the decision to remain sober and still have a great time. It may take a while to develop healthy habits, but they'll vastly improve your life.

The Habit Chaining technique is quite effective for folks with AUD. Introduced by the *Wall Street Journal* bestselling author, S.J Scott, the premise is that making small life changes in your habits has quite an impact. "Build routines around habits that don't require effort" because "small wins build momentum. They're easy to remember and complete," stated Scott in his 2014 book, *Habit Stacking: 97 Small Life Changes That Take Five Minutes or Less*. He proposed the theory of "habit chaining," describing it as a process of grouping together small activities into routine behaviors that ultimately give rise to a new habit.

The "reward" is the next step in solidifying a healthy habit you've just created. When drinking is replaced with a new pattern, the reward you perceive in having a drink plays a vital role in the process. Say the happy hour drink is fun not just because of the booze buzz but also because you're hanging out with friends and you can let loose. You can still experience the same camaraderie if you have a non-alcoholic drink instead. The new habit you're creating could be anything, and the reward, too, can be anything you enjoy. Dissect what gives you pleasure and focus on what truly feels rewarding to you.

Remember, the key to developing any good habit is to be consistent with it. Be determined to achieve the reward you deserve and work toward it. Change might be slow at first, but the marginal gains will sustain you in the long run. The power of marginal gains in sobriety plays a significant role in recovery.

Achieving incremental goals is all about the small details. If you're working on sobriety, an incremental goal could include taking care of, say, your teeth. Since alcohol affects the health of your gums, you might lose your teeth relatively earlier in life. Alcohol also gives you bad breath, so there's another reason to quit. An adjunct benefit of stopping drinking is having fresh breath. You're now considering improved oral hygiene in general. Good oral hygiene is now a part of your life and, before you know it, this will extend to overall self-care. Why would you just limit concern about your body to oral hygiene? You also want to have good skin, which is connected to eating a healthy diet, exercise, stress-free days, and more. This is the essence of a healthy lifestyle—good habits.

Once you get into the healthy zone, set a date on your calendar a year from now. That's the day you anticipate proudly announcing your sobriety. Focus on that date, and each time it gets tough, take a look at next year's calendar and remain determined to achieve your quest. You know you can do it.

Detox and Withdrawal

Alcohol affects the body at a cellular level, which results in the dysfunction of the brain's neurochemicals. The neurochemicals become imbalanced, which can be seen shortly after someone has a drink. The withdrawal symptoms, too, are the result of this imbalance. The "withdrawal syndrome" occurs when an individual with AUD abstains from drinking alcohol. Once your body has become addicted to alcohol, the brain's main inhibitory chemical, GABA, and its main excitatory chemical, glutamate, become dysfunctional. The brain's function relies heavily on the coordinated transmission of GABA and glutamate signals. These two neurotransmitters are responsible for many functions. GABA plays a role in how we experience anxiety, fear, and stress. And Glutamate is associated with memory and learning. Impaired uptake of glutamate is associated with stroke, autism, some forms of intellectual disability, and diseases such as amyotrophic lateral sclerosis and Alzheimer's disease.

Alcohol acts like a sedative, stimulating the body to

release more GABA. GABA blocks signals and results in a slowdown in brain and nervous system activity. This means alcohol hinders your cognition, affects your memory and attentiveness, and even gets in the way of your ability to interact with people and situations.

The way alcohol affects the nervous system results in acute withdrawal symptoms that can be fatal. Binge drinkers, in particular, are at risk of extreme withdrawal symptoms, which is why heavy indulgers need to check with a doctor when they try to get sober. The first 14 days of abstinence will be the hardest because of something called "the kick." If you can get through the first 14 days, everything gets easier. Withdrawal symptoms commonly affect adult binge drinkers, but teenagers or younger individuals with AUD can also experience the effects. The symptoms are challenging but can be treated. Therefore, professional supervision is necessary.

The alcohol withdrawal process involves the following three stages:

Stage 1: The first six to 12 hours of alcohol detox. This is when you'll likely experience headache, nausea, stomach ache, and insomnia.

Stage 2: The next 12 to 48 hours. This is when symptoms can become scary. Some people even experience seizures and hallucinations.

Stage 3: The last 48 to 72 hours, which are the hardest. An individual may suffer a racing heartbeat, high blood pressure, delirium tremens, sweating, fever, confusion, auditory hallucinations, and, potentially, death.

These withdrawal symptoms can send the brain's neurotransmitters into shock because, as we've mentioned, alcohol affects the body on a cellular level, so the entire body is affected. This is precisely why you need to be under a professional's care when detoxing. Your age, weight, the intensity of the addiction, and other health issues must be considered when developing your detox plan. Doctors and other healthcare professionals can help you through the detox and withdrawal stages with the assistance of medications like beta-blockers, anti-anxiety drugs, or other pharmaceuticals.

Apart from all that, attempting to detox at home is almost always ineffective when dealing with the kick. The urge to resume drinking will be strong, and many tend to give in. A boot camp or rehab facility is much more effective in helping an individual to effectively and safely achieve sobriety. As mentioned earlier, you may experience setbacks, but trying to stop drinking at home—when you have alcohol in your fridge, or you can easily drive to the store to get it—is a recipe for failure.

Chapter 4 – The Approach

"It does not matter how slowly you go, only that you do not stop." — Confucius

Ironically, a dangerous substance like alcohol is still legal to purchase and use in most parts of the world. "Not everyone who drinks is an alcoholic," they say, but assuredly, anyone who drinks may be at risk of becoming one. The question is, why take that chance in the first place? If there's nothing more precious than life, why do we tempt fate as we do by risking harming ourselves? It only makes sense that anything that puts your life at risk should be avoided entirely, yet our collective societies foster alcoholism to a certain extent.

Treating AUD saves lives, and finding out the root cause of the addiction is a revelation in the process. This book focuses on four core aspects involved in alcoholism: addiction, biological, psychological, and social. Addressing these four core factors will allow you to build a rock-solid foundation from which you can enjoy a life of sobriety for years to come. You must completely embrace each principle if you seek long-term success. One of the primary overarching ideas is fully committing to recovery in all areas of your life. All of these factors work together. It's unlikely that you'll achieve lasting success with sobriety without addressing all of them.

Principle 1: Addiction

Alcoholism is a progressive disorder, and prolonged alcohol abuse takes a toll on your health in many ways. The earlier the problem is detected and addressed, the better for your health and your life. As mentioned earlier, the first step in the recovery process—after acknowledging you have a problem—is detox. With the difficult initial phase of detox accomplished, you'll encounter the second-hand challenges of abstinence. The entire approach to sobriety comes into question when triggers become strong. Sticking to your commitment is the only way through.

Managing triggers is what sobriety is all about. The question is, how do we do that? A personalized approach will help you control your triggers. There's always a reason behind an urge, be it your body's biological response to a stimulus or the external environment or circumstances that instigate the trigger. The following points will help you narrow down the reasons behind your motivations.

Emotional episodes

Being an AUD sufferer is hard enough. It's a constant battle. Gaining the courage to face the truth that you have AUD and start working on improving yourself are huge milestones. Some people may have to stop communicating with friends and family for prolonged periods to stay strong in this process. This can temporarily take a toll on an individual's mental health, which may already be compromised by many years of alcohol abuse. There may come a point when emotions are overpowering and trigger the urge the drink. When this happens, it's essential to know you can ignore the trigger and distract yourself from what's stressing you out.

Over-thinking

When you're in recovery, chemicals in your body fluctuate and make you feel you're on a roller-coaster of emotions and physical effects. This may eventually lead you to over-thinking your decision to abstain, and you may even consider abandoning your effort. This is all a part of your recovery, so don't give in to your doubts and rationalizations. Feelings of hopelessness and negativity can sometimes arise regardless of your personal problems. It's not you; it's a symptom of the recovery process. Stay strong.

Trauma

Trauma is a significant part of human life, and it can

be one of the largest contributors to mental health problems, including depression, anxiety, and addiction. According to the National Council for Behavioral Health, 70% of adults in the United States have experienced at least one traumatic event, which means that 223 million people in the US alone have had trauma. Moreover, among people who seek treatment for mental health issues, 90% have gone through trauma.

Time doesn't necessarily heal all wounds. It merely allows them to fade into the background to make it easier for you to go through the day. The days eventually become easier, but the wound may never fully be healed, depending on the situation. And that's okay. Some scars will never truly fade, and it's normal to be haunted by certain experiences. You don't have to get down on yourself for being emotionally caught up in the past sometimes. Trauma and tragedy are part of our lives.

When rehab and seclusion are part of your effort to get sober, traumas can sometimes resurface and upset you. In fact, don't be surprised if a past trauma is reignited to a greater extent during your days of recovery. This is why talking to a counselor is an essential part of the process. Triggers that you previously attempted to deal with by drinking will arise, so you need help to create new habits for dealing with unpleasant thoughts and memories.

Your External Environment

There will be times when even a certain atmosphere will have you craving alcohol. It could be a meal you used to enjoy with a particular wine or even music that you always listened to with a drink in your hand. Smells, tastes, sounds, places, and even the weather may trigger your urge, but you're on the road to recovery, so recognize these environmental triggers for what they are, and don't give in.

If you do give in, look at what triggered you and vow not to let that happen again. Even if it was a full-blown relapse, don't be discouraged. The cells in your body aren't under your command, and almost everyone pursuing sobriety has relapsed at least once. A relapse is always a possibility, so be prepared for it. What matters is that there's no reason it should prevent you from achieving your goal.

Principle 2: Biological

Your physical health plays a crucial role in sobriety. Sleep, nutrition, and fitness are essential factors in maintaining and sustaining a sober lifestyle. Individuals suffering from AUD are prone to a deficiency of B-complex vitamins such as thiamine, folate or folic acid, and B12. There may also be a vitamin C deficiency. Meals rich in carbohydrates can help restore your body to health. Pasta, bread, potatoes, carrots, beans, legumes, and lentils combined with protein can help reverse the effects of alcoholism.

Principle 3: Psychological

This principle focuses on your psychological health, which includes self-confidence, spirituality, and emotional well-being. Sobriety is a long journey, and a significant part of it involves removing yourself from aspects of your previous life. Boot camps and rehab facilities are located away from cities so that residents can get in touch with their true self, free from distractions. Sobriety means recreating your lifestyle, which doesn't just mean removing alcohol from your bloodstream but also purifying your headspace.

Meditating and focusing on your mental health play a vital role in recovery. Beneficial psychological factors will sustain you in the long run. Developing a daily routine that keeps you productive and busy with meaningful work has helped many AUD sufferers. A positive outlook on life is what sobriety promotes, and an individual starting recovery needs to make sure they embrace this idea to the fullest.

Principle 4: Social

This principle focuses on helping you identify, improve, and develop the right kinds of social relationships in your life during recovery and beyond. Social constructs and relationships play such a massive role in our everyday life, and they strongly support or damage our chances of a successful recovery.

An AUD sufferer needs to find a way to navigate each social setting in which drinking is involved. You need to learn how to say no to an offer of alcohol without feeling uncomfortable. It takes practice, but you'll soon be able to participate in a variety of social settings and remain sober. However, individuals in recovery need to ensure their social environment supports their recovery.

Chapter 5 – Addiction Focus

A Brief History of Addiction

Although this book is primarily dedicated to helping you in your journey to freedom from alcohol addiction, we fully acknowledge the many other forms of addiction that have crippled generations and led individuals to poverty, illness, and early death. Addiction predates the recorded history of the Egyptian and Roman empires, but it wasn't until the advent of agriculture and farming that it became more common. Centuries later, a massive number of people around the world have become addicted to a variety of substances.

Approximately 13,000 years ago, farmers grew addictive substances like marijuana, opium, and others. Because they could produce these substances in large quantities, addiction witnessed a rise. Although plant-based addictive substances were relatively easy to produce, in early times, their market was limited to specific areas since certain plants could only grow on a particular type of soil. In the 1800s, the world advanced into the science of chemistry and pharmaceuticals. The advent of international trade allowed addictive substances such as amphetamine (1887), ecstasy (1912), PCP (1926), ketamine (1962), and other illicit drugs to be sold easily around the world

Substance abuse isn't new. What's alarming is that the rate of addiction continues to increase, and newer, more powerful, and more dangerous substances are available. Some drugs can now induce zombie-like behavior in humans, and some drugs have drastic, long-term effects on the body. Addiction is a dilemma of modern society, and substance abuse is often part of the lifestyle of celebrities and other famous figures, with alcoholism still being one of its most popular forms.

The Addiction Cycle

The American Society of Addiction Medicine defines addiction as a chronic disorder that takes a toll on the abuser's memory, motivations, and ability to feel pleasure and reward. Alcoholism is a progressive disease in which emotions, behavior, and genetics may cause a person to move from a few drinks a night to binge drinking to the use of other addictive substances.

Addiction develops in stages. The cycle of addiction is similar whether the abused substance is alcohol or an illicit drug. Just as with alcohol, the body develops tolerance to a drug, which means greater and greater quantities are required to achieve the same level of effect. The goal is to break this cycle. To accomplish that, you must first be aware of the stages:

- Initial use
- Abuse

- Tolerance
- Dependence
- Addiction
- Relapse

Recovery endorses a bottom-up approach to break the cycle. Seeking treatment at a dedicated rehab facility reduces the chances of relapse, weans your body off the addictive substance, reduces your dependence on alcohol or the illicit drug(s), and strengthens your resolve, so your life of abuse becomes history.

Fighting Addiction Is Hard

Individuals with AUD could spend years not knowing they have a problem. Even when they face it, fighting the addiction is a considerable challenge. Nonetheless, the cycle can be interrupted, and professional treatment has helped saved lives. Treatment in a rehab facility or with the help of a professional is the surest way to success. Alcohol recovery teams use protocols developed through scientific research. The amount of research on alcoholism has done wonders in the fight against it.

There are multiple forms of treatment available for alcoholism. Cognitive-behavioral therapy has been shown to play a significant role in helping individuals break out of the cycle of addiction. Psychological problems stem from numerous causes, with faulty thinking patterns playing a significant role. These patterns develop subconsciously under unfavorable circumstances like a family history of alcohol or drug abuse, childhood neglect and abuse, depression, loneliness, social issues, a difficult home environment when the individual is growing up, and peer/family pressure. Cognitive-behavioral therapy targets the thinking patterns that lead a person to seek refuge in alcohol. It highlights the faults in an individual's perception of a given circumstance and allows them to see things differently. This type of therapy eventually rewires an individual's distorted patterns and unhelpful behavior, enabling them to effectively tackle challenging scenarios rather than resorting to drinking. Other forms of adjunctive treatment for addiction include peer support groups, medication, and physical therapy.

Setting a Quit Date

Sobriety focuses on anticipating dates an individual sets as benchmarks in their recovery. Each of these dates is celebrated, and this is a strong motivational factor for an AUD sufferer. Clean dates or sobriety dates are milestones commemorating success and celebrating another chance at life. These milestones could include the date a person quits drinking, the date they enroll in rehab, or the date they've gone a month without a drink.

A sobriety date will let an individual with AUD set a time frame and track their journey to note their progress and be less likely to relapse. Keeping track of the days of sobriety is a powerful part of a successful rehab.

Although setting a quit date is regarded as a crucial factor in achieving recovery, some have argued that setting a quit date can be detrimental to the addict. Long-time 12-step critic Stanton Peele has argued that sobriety dates or clean dates instill feelings of shame and failure in those who relapse. A change of mindset is needed in this regard. To begin with, what other people say or think doesn't matter when it comes to questions of life and death. A sobriety date should be considered a milestone to help keep you on track. If you relapse, you keep going forward with your recovery. As long as you hold the mindset of working on staying sober, you're a step ahead of who you were yesterday. It's a slow and steady process, and dates serve to record your progress.

Identifying and Managing Triggers

Triggers fall under two categories—external and internal. Succumbing to a trigger can severely impact an individual's recovery, regardless of its nature. Examples of a few triggers are:

- Depression
- Fear
- Grief
- Stress
- PTSD
- Abuse
- Feelings of unworthiness, shame, or guilt

Apart from the triggers mentioned above, there may be specific triggers that make you susceptible to relapse, but if you have a strong resolve, you can resist. Managing triggers is all about self-awareness. The moment you feel triggered to resort to your old ways of coping, question yourself about what the result will be if you do that. Will alcohol cure the problem or make the trigger less painful? It certainly won't. Will drinking help you find a solution to your discomfort? No, it won't. Does it harm you if you don't react to the trigger by drinking? No, it doesn't. Identify what's triggering you and try to step out of your current environment or distract yourself in a healthy way. Better yet, talk to a counselor about your triggers so you're ready to deal with them when they arise. A counselor can help you manage triggers, and eventually, you won't respond to them anymore. Exercise, getting enough sleep, joining a support group, meditation, and recreational activities can also help you manage triggers more effectively. Triggers can be overcome, so don't give in to them.

Recognizing Relapse Warning Signs

Relapse has been categorized into three aspects: emotional, mental, and physical. A relapse can happen anytime during your recovery phase, and the worst part of it is emotional rather than physical. It doesn't harm your body to the degree it harms your motivation. The road to relapse begins long before you pick up a drink. A relapse can sneak up on you, usually because you don't recognize the warning signs.

Emotional Relapse

This is the most debilitating of the three aspects and, during this phase, you'll find yourself struggling with the following:

- Staying secluded or away from situations that may trigger you to drink
- Not attending your scheduled recovery meetings and activities
- Failing to look after yourself
- Poor eating and sleeping habits
- Mood swings

- Intolerance
- Paying more attention to others to avoid your problems
- An overall attitude of not caring about anything
- Defensiveness
- Not accepting help

These symptoms need immediate attention. Journaling about your recovery each day is a practical and effective approach to warding off a relapse. Deep breathing, meditating, and creating more positivity in your environment will help you snap out any dark thoughts and get you back on track.

Mental Relapse

When you turn a blind eye to an emotional relapse, chances are you'll fall prey to the second aspect of relapse, which is the mental component. Best described as a war within oneself, a person undergoing mental relapse takes on a dual personality: a person who wants to drink and a person who opposes the idea. An individual may enter an almost trance-like state, fantasizing about their escape from the commitment they made. The mental relapse aspect challenges the individual to the core and increases their vulnerability. The symptoms of mental relapse may include:

- Reverting to old habits in general
- Hanging out with friends who drink
- Reminiscing to others about past experiences with alcohol or drugs and boasting about it
- Lying
- Bargaining for why it's okay to have a drink: "It's the holidays."
- Switching to other forms of substance abuse to alleviate the urge somehow
- Fantasizing about a relapse
- Trying to escape the recovery process
- Missing out on scheduled meetings

Urges can last between 10 to 30 minutes, so stay put for at least that long. Think about the consequences of what will happen if you give in. Think about all the determination, suffering, and cost you've endured to come this far. Think about the worry you'd cause your loved ones. Is one drink worth all that? Talk it over with a peer who understands what you're going through. Be open about your thoughts and fears. Seek help and remember: You've made it this far without a drink, so you can keep moving forward in your sobriety.

Physical Relapse

When a person doesn't take the time to acknowledge and address the symptoms of emotional and mental relapse, it doesn't take long before physical relapse occurs. This includes the act of drinking alcohol or using one's preferred drug of choice.

Taking one drink can be considered a "lapse" or slip-up. Physical relapse is a return to uncontrollable use. If this happens, some people will continue to use for months, while others realize what they've done and stop much sooner, returning their focus to recovery.

After relapsing, specific steps can be taken to get yourself back on the right track. Experts recommend that those in recovery think about situations in which they'll have the opportunity to use and rehearse what they'll do to prevent another relapse.

Chapter 6 – Biological Focus

Food and water are the building blocks of life. When it comes to recovery, food plays a vital role in restoring your body's health. Some foods can even reverse the debilitating effects of alcoholism. Once you've embarked on the road to recovery, specific changes occur inside your body. Your body begins healing during the detox stage, and the alcohol-free lifestyle requires some significant changes in what you feast on. Your immune system has been compromised by ingesting alcohol, and that means you need to eat a balanced diet that will supplement your body with the right kind of nutrients.

In the initial days of detox, vomiting and feeling sick will be the norm. You likely won't have much appetite for food, but don't be alarmed. This is a normal part of the process. A poor appetite is only temporary. Nonetheless, you still need to eat a healthy diet during the initial stage as you wait for your appetite to return. Long-term AUD may cause deficiencies of vitamins in your body, and recovery focuses extensively on replenishing those deficiencies.

Nutrition

Nutrition is the foundation of your physical health. Addiction can impact your physical body in many ways depending on what you're addicted to, but side effects can include:

- Depletion of specific vital nutrients such as B vitamins (B1, B6, and folic acid)
- Damage to the liver and kidneys
- Imbalance of protein, electrolytes, fluids, and calories
- Weight loss and malnutrition
- Mistaking feelings of hunger for cravings

Perhaps the most telling thing about nutrition is its impact on your mental well-being. Food plays a crucial role in helping us to feel good. According to the Mental Health Foundation, proper dietary choices are directly associated with higher levels of mental well-being. Eating a healthy diet is a smart way to build a base from which healing can begin.

The five aspects of a healthy diet plan must include the following:

1. Keep Yourself Hydrated

Sufficient daily water intake is always crucial, but this becomes especially important when detoxing from alcohol addiction. A cleansing of the body begins with assuring you're drinking plenty of water. Ironically, although alcohol is a beverage, it dehydrates the body. It's a diuretic, and once it enters your bloodstream, it flushes out essential nutrients through the renal system. A diuretic causes the kidneys to flush fluids from your body at a faster rate, and if you've been an AUD sufferer for long, you need to replenish your body's fluid levels.

Once you're in detox, your body will begin to flush out toxins, and vomiting and diarrhea are the most extreme detox effects. This is why drinking plenty of water is essential.

2. Vegetables and Fruits

Studies have described a decrease in folate and vitamin A in individuals with prolonged alcohol abuse. Vegetables can allow an individual to feel full without the extra calories, and fruits are a healthier alternative to sugary cocktails that the individual with AUD is accustomed to. Alcohol detox often induces cravings for sweets, and fruits will trick the mind into getting what it's demanding minus the alcohol. Experts believe foods high in sugar stimulate the brain the same way alcohol does. A can of soda will do the same, but what's the point of removing one type of chemical from your body to replace it with another? Eating something natural is the way to go. Nutritionists advise opting for whole fruits instead of fruit juices.

3. Protein

Alcohol attacks protein molecules in particular, so people suffering from AUD can develop a protein deficiency. Ethyl alcohol denatures protein, so it's essential that people who have a history of alcoholism eat enough protein. Protein builds and maintains muscle. A lack of protein can have dire consequences, including fatigue, decreased strength, loss of muscle mass, and increased risk of bone fractures. Poultry, fish, peas, beans, legumes, nuts, and vitamin E-rich foods should be incorporated into your diet during alcohol detox. Magnesium, iron, and zinc levels should be checked as well.

4. Whole Grains

Carbohydrate deficiency is common in individuals with AUD. Alcohol facilitates the esterification of carbohydrates, which can lead to hypoglycemia. Carbs are a great source of fiber and calories, which the AUD sufferer often doesn't eat enough of. Sobriety is all about a clean body, which means eating healthy, unrefined foods. Make sure your carbs are nutritionally complete rather than processed grains.

Whole grains like quinoa, brown bread, and oats are rich in vitamin B and a great source of carbohydrates.

5. Savory Soups

Sobriety certainly doesn't mean that when you stop drinking alcohol you have permission to eat anything you want. Detoxing your body is all about staying fit, active, and refraining from consuming harmful substances. Alcohol is poisonous for your body, so since you've decided to stop drinking to improve your health, you need to avoid unhealthy, processed food.

Soups are a great way to go when detoxing, especially if you're dealing with nausea, indigestion, and vomiting. Be sure the soups are prepared from scratch with no artificial ingredients.

A balanced diet will sustain your body through the recovery phase and facilitate its healing from alcoholism. Keep in mind that detoxing from alcohol is hard on your body, so you need to treat it well during the process. Detoxing will often make you lose your appetite and lose weight, so you must replenish lost nutrients.

Fitness and Exercise

The word "fitness" strikes fear into the hearts and minds of many people. Our conscious and subconscious minds still remember those difficult physical education classes at school. As adults, we're expected to carry on a physically active lifestyle on our own. Thanks to an industry built around making people feel bad about their appearance, we've lost the understanding of what it means to be fit.

For those in recovery, we need to adjust this definition. Fitness can be a truly powerful force in both maintaining and enjoying sobriety. It can be tempting to only think of fitness as something you do to try and lose a few pounds or get those six-pack abs. However, fitness should be thought of not as just a means of achieving some physical benefit but as something that nourishes your entire being.

Ground-breaking discoveries about the beneficial effects of exercise and fitness have taken the detox process to a whole other level of success. Engaging in exercise modifies the brain's pathways and rewires the reward system, which can turn things around for the AUD sufferer. Exercising releases endorphins, the feel-good chemicals in the body, so you have a sense of joy following a good workout. Exercise can also increase your energy level and improve sleep quality..

Withdrawing from alcohol isn't just a war that takes place in one's mind but also in the physical body. Vomiting and diarrhea cause a person to feel drained and low on energy, so start slow during your recovery with short walks outdoors. As the days pass, the individual should implement a workout routine at a gym or other setting. Focusing on the body makes it easier to deal with the urge to drink.

Sleep

Pulling yourself through a significant illness like alcoholism isn't just about a change of lifestyle but a change of the body as well. You'll feel and see the difference in yourself as you get healthier, which means you've transitioned into a new and improved you. Although this may not be as evident in your appearance, the transition has a considerable impact from a psychological perspective.

In this regard, sleep plays a significant role. Rest heals the body. When it comes to the emotional stress of withdrawal, sleep is crucial. From preventing dementia to inhibiting the development of diabetes, adequate, good-quality sleep is essential.

The symptoms of withdrawal from alcohol affect sleep patterns significantly. During the first week of detox, people often experience insomnia. Individuals may fall asleep easily but wake up in the middle of the night feeling agitated. Some might find it hard to sleep and may report their sleep isn't restorative. Disrupted sleep patterns are what cause a majority of AUD sufferers to relapse.

Alcohol works its magic by putting an individual into a quick, deep state of slumber. This is precisely why many people with depression or anxiety resort to alcohol. Most withdrawal symptoms resolve over time, but sleep disorders take longer to fix. The Substance

Abuse and Mental Health Services Administration (SAMHSA) stated that 25% to 72% of people with alcohol use disorder report sleep troubles. In recovery, cognitive behavioral therapy for insomnia (CBT-I) may be helpful to an individual having difficulty sleeping. Other treatment options include medication, aromatherapy, spiritual healing, and more.

Fueling Your Body's Capacity to Heal

A combination of diet, exercise, sleep, and mindfulness will work wonders in assuring you stay on the path of sobriety. Nonetheless, breaking free from AUD requires professional help that includes therapy and, often, medication. A rehab facility keeps track of all aspects of your physical well-being, from your health history to the current state of your body. Blood work and examinations will reveal any areas of concern, so any necessary action is taken in a timely manner. Supplements and a good diet may be all that's needed for some individuals, while others may need more intensive treatment if alcohol has damaged their vital organs.

The point is, everyone is unique, and not every AUD sufferer will have the same signs and symptoms. A personalized approach is needed to fuel the body to maximize its healing capacity. Connecting with a dietician is a proactive approach in creating a healthier lifestyle when detoxing and afterward. A diet plan can be designed to meet your needs. Alternatively, seek a peer group that's involved in nutrition education to help you create a diet plan.

A newbie in recovery may sometimes feel ill just at the sight of food. Small and healthy meals consumed four or five times a day can help build your tolerance for and interest in eating. Under a professional's care, you'll find ways to deal with these side effects of recovery. What must take priority is making sure your diet consists of a range of healthy foods and plenty of water.

Chapter 7 – Psychological Focus

Mastering Your Mental Health

There's a tendency in most cultures to avoid discussing our mental health with others, and therefore it's become a taboo subject. We hold things in and mask our true feelings, which creates stress over time. These withheld feelings and thoughts can impair our decision-making abilities. As someone in recovery, developing your ability to make good decisions is crucial.

If you encounter a potential relapse trigger while

holding onto bottled-up emotions, you might not be able to think clearly or rationally. Being in control of your thoughts, feelings, and beliefs may be a novel idea. Your mental health requires ongoing attention and care throughout your life. It protects and provides the control you need, especially in recovery when the goal is long-term sobriety.

Addiction might have taken control of your life without you being aware it was happening, but if you've made it this far reading this book, you now understand that addiction is curable. With the power of your mind, you can overcome it. The good news is, you don't have to do any of this alone. Depression, anxiety, and other mental health issues are a part of everyone's life, but in patients with AUD, these are more prevalent. From outpatient help to inpatient treatment, you can obtain professional help when you're faced with psychological troubles while you're going through withdrawal.

A guaranteed hack to sustain a healthy mindset is to realize you're improving your life every day you don't drink. Many of your worries will cease, and each passing day brings you closer to your destiny.

Substance abuse is curable, and you're already on your way to recovery. What was driving you to alcoholism is no longer in charge. The worst is behind you, and you're well along your journey when you decide to get sober. Don't let a disorder define your life.

Living Intentionally

For some, "living intentionally" means having a clear intention for every action. In alcohol recovery, living intentionally means having a proactive approach in which the primary motive is to improve your health mentally, emotionally, and physically. Looking after the body requires attention to physical needs like food, water, and sleep. A considerable part of intentional living is the firm belief in the value of living in the present moment and setting goals. It also promotes kindness, empathy, and being grateful for the blessings in our life.

Living intentionally is particularly helpful in recovery because it can help prevent an individual from having a relapse. Setting small goals for each day—especially if it's a bad day—helps prevent individuals from bouncing back into their old habits.

For example, consider this scenario: Lisa is 16, and she had a bad day at school. She was made fun of, and the guy she likes asked another girl out. The teacher scolded her for not paying attention, and she felt embarrassed. When she got home, she changed into her pajamas and binge-watched Friends episodes until she dozed off. The following day, Lisa got up and went to school feeling much better. On the other hand, Bill is 48, and he was picked on at work. The manager seemed to find fault with everything he did. He had a heated argument with the manager and left his job early to try to switch off his brain, just as Lisa did when she watched all those episodes of Friends. Since Bill has AUD, he went straight to the liquor store and bought two six-packs of beer. He went home and drank until he passed out.

If Bill had lived intentionally that day, he wouldn't have resorted to drinking. Every action should have a clear intention of living with purpose. Binge drinking has no purpose whatsoever, and that's where Bill would have drawn the line had he lived intentionally.

He didn't set small goals for his day—like staying at the office until his usual time to leave, going home and opening up about his day to his wife, having dinner with his family, and then dozing off to wake up with a clear head for the next day at work.

Living intentionally lets individuals take steps that will benefit their mental health and contribute to their sense of contentment. It diminishes behaviors that harm the body and can help eliminate procrastination and unhealthy thinking patterns.

Prioritize Wellness and Self-care

Self-care is one of the most important aspects of recovery. Active alcohol use may have left you neglecting yourself and your basic needs. As an alcoholic, you might have spent days in bed. Poor hygiene, an unbalanced diet, and a deteriorating social life are all repercussions of self-neglect. In recovery, you do the opposite. The cardinal principle of healing is to prioritize yourself and take care of your needs no matter what. Some might think this sounds selfish, but when it's AUD we're talking about, self-love is crucial.

Small acts of self-care like taking a long warm shower, buying yourself something you like, meditation, and adequate sleep help alleviate stress and make your recovery easier. The neglect your body endured while you were under the influence of alcohol needs to be reversed. While medications and detox take care of you from the inside, acts of kindness to yourself and mindfulness will take care of you from the outside. Only you can pull yourself through, so give yourself plenty of love and caring.

Positive Mindset

The idea of having a positive mindset in recovery is often misconstrued. Being positive doesn't mean you have to put on a bright face even when you feel like dying on the inside. A positive mindset has to do with your thought process. It means continually focusing on the positive side of things rather than the negative. Being an AUD sufferer is a grim situation, but there's a cure, so focus on the treatment. Asking for help is a positive gesture, while keeping your addiction bottled inside or neglecting it won't help you.

A positive mindset will make the recovery phase a lot smoother. Believing in yourself and knowing you deserve every bit of love and attention you receive—from yourself or others—is what positivity is about. Even if you relapse, stay positive and know it's all a part of the game. When the going gets tough, believe that you'll come out stronger. Believe in yourself, and keep going.

Affirmations

Never underestimate the power of words. Hurtful words spoken to us can stay with us forever. Words have brought about revolutions and have destroyed whole communities. When in recovery, the power of words intensifies. Affirmations are an extension of the positive mindset we mentioned earlier. Reciting or reading affirmations is a practice that destroys discouragement and negativity.

Words we tell our self often have a more significant impact than what someone else tells us. In recovery, negative thoughts and feelings are an impediment. The science of affirmations endorses the same ideology. A study published in the journal *Social Cognitive and Affective Neuroscience* used MRI to reveal the impact of words on the reward centers in the brain. Repeating positive phrases like, "I deserve a better life" or "One step at a time" will help activate the brain's reward centers, augmenting the motivation an individual in recovery needs.

Other positive phrases or affirmations that are empowering include:

- "I love myself."
- "I'm enough to make myself happy."
- "Progress doesn't mean I have to be perfect."
- "I'll never give up."
- "I believe I can do this.

Managing Stress

Stress plays a significant role in relapse, and that's precisely why managing stress takes top priority in rehab. Stress isn't avoidable but it's manageable. From minor issues like being late for school to more major problems like a bad relationship, stress can take a toll on your life even when you're sober. The following methods will help you manage stress better:

- Meditation: Meditation allows you to witness your thoughts and be able to see beyond the stressful situation to the bigger picture. It gives you a bird's eye view and creates distance between you and your problem, allowing you to view it more clearly. It may even enable you to find a solution to what's causing you stress.

- Let it out: Be it crying or just opening up about your worries with a professional or a peer, talking out your feelings lets you process the stress and view a situation from a different perspective. It allows you to think out of the box and understand that whatever is stressing you out will pass, and you'll pull through.

- Socialize: Stepping out of your usual surroundings for a while and catching up with friends and family can expand your perspective and be a great de-stressor. You'll gain insight into their lives and situations and realize you're not the only one facing stressful events. A little diversion and light-hearted laughter benefits just about anyone. Just make sure your drinks aren't a part of your socializing.

Willpower

Without willpower, sobriety is pretty much an illusion. Although willpower alone can't help you attain sobriety, it plays a vital role. Scientific studies define willpower as:

- The ability to restrain oneself from engaging in negative actions
- The ability to control one's urges
- The dedication to sustain one self through rough patches in life
- Self-discipline
- The ability to stay steadfast against temptations to achieve greater rewards

In recovery, willpower is necessary to both attain and sustain the sobriety you're striving to achieve. An individual with AUD will face countless temptations to relapse. Willpower is required, and if it's strong enough, nothing can stop you from reaching your goals.

Avoiding Temptation

When you're in the initial phases of recovery, you need to minimize stress, drama, temptations, and every factor that can trigger you into relapsing. Going out with your drinking buddies or frequenting restaurants and eateries that feature alcohol is a no-no for the abstainer. Do yourself a favor and eliminate anything in your life that will make it harder for you to abstain. Explore new places to meet friends, eat, and have fun where alcohol isn't available. You'll soon find out there are many more ways of enjoying yourself than just getting drunk.

This may be the perfect opportunity to expand your horizons and explore new cultures, cuisines, and entertainment that don't include drinking. Yes, there are places in the world where alcohol isn't a part of anything. Meeting new people and learning more about their culture and norms will help you gain a bigger perspective on life, allowing you to understand how limiting a life that's fueled by alcohol can be.

Journaling

Journaling about your recovery is a great way to reflect on your achievements. Don't worry if you haven't completed any of the tasks you set for yourself on a particular day. You can still write down your thoughts and feelings, and you'll see the difference it makes. Psychologists believe journaling brings clarity to the mind and encourages awareness of your deepest thoughts and motivations. In the process of writing, you might feel like breaking down and crying, which is a step toward emotional recovery. You might even come up with a solution to something you're stressed about or have been trying to figure out. This will reveal your true inner wisdom and allow you to value yourself all the more.

Journaling is a personal record that you can use to track your recovery as well as something to reflect on. It's an act of self-care that helps you focus on your capabilities, your flaws, and the solutions at hand. It's also an act of self-mastery, and since recovery has much to do with mastering your willpower, journaling plays a vital role.

Chapter 8 – Social Focus

We live in an age obsessed with socializing and being popular. Loners are often looked upon as odd, dysfunctional creatures who relish their life of solitude. Although keeping to oneself is a good idea at times, it's not a healthy situation in the long run. Family bonds and friends are what life is about. Just as social settings can lead you down the path to alcoholism, the right kind of social setting can help you recover from it, too.

Family and friends give meaning to life. They make life worth fighting for, but that certainly doesn't mean you should undermine your sense of self-worth to help or please another. It's true that you're complete and sufficient for your own happiness, but this doesn't provide the same satisfaction you feel when you can celebrate your life with the ones you love. Humans are built to be social creatures, so we must take care of our social needs. Nonetheless, your social circle can, at times, interfere with your quest for sobriety. Let's explore this in detail.

Family and Friends

Speaking, thinking, and positive journaling may be in your control—and these can certainly contribute significantly to your recovery—but what about the factors in your life that you have no control over? Friends, family, and relationships are a part of life—and perhaps what makes life feel complete—but what if those closest to us sabotage our recovery?

Alcoholism is everywhere, and chances are, you aren't the only one you know struggling with the disorder—although you might be one of only a few seeking sobriety. The sad truth is that most AUD sufferers don't want to face their problem and won't seek help.

An individual with AUD typically has a family background in which at least one other individual has the same problem.

At times, there will be people around you who don't support your sobriety or will actively try to sabotage it. They could be a member of your close family or a friend next door. In situations in which you feel like someone is interfering with your efforts to get sober, you can try the following:

- Avoid hanging out with that person if they encourage you to share a drink with them.
- Learn to say no. Politely excuse yourself from situations that may trigger a relapse.
- Come up with an exit plan to leave when a situation gets too "drunk" around you.
- Don't listen to people who are skeptical about your ability to get sober.
- Be patient with people who find the new you to be a stranger. It will take time for the people around you to adapt to your calmer personality.

Professional Relationships

In the professional world, you'll have to face similar situations. Unfortunately, professional environments are some of the most challenging for those who are trying to recover from an addiction or are now sober. Whether you're in school or have a career, your addiction has undoubtedly made an impact on where you are today. How you approach and handle your professional relationships can help or hinder your future success.

There's no one-size-fits-all approach when dealing with relationships at school and work. You need to learn how to read the room and understand your current situation. At some point, you'll have to decide if and how you want talk about your addiction in a professional setting. You'll need a backup plan, and you also need to learn how to distance yourself from toxic coworkers or classmates.

You might also need to know when talking to someone higher up is necessary and how to tell if you should start searching for a new job. Thinking through all these scenarios can feel overwhelming. However, if you're prepared and have thought through most potential situations, you can safely navigate the professional world while avoiding issues relating to recovery and sobriety.

For example, your boss may believe that drinking is an essential social activity and, as an authority figure, they might not accept your recovery and try to intimidate you into having a drink. The best way to handle situations like this is to say no politely. You might have to attend a business dinner, and you may be asked to make a toast. You can still make a toast and pretend to drink without actually doing so, thereby maintaining your professional relationship while not sabotaging your sobriety.

There's always a safe zone in the middle somewhere, and all you have to do is find your way to it. Opening up to work colleagues about your struggles isn't professional. Staying diplomatic yet firm in your convictions is the way to go. Don't make a point of how you aren't drinking but simply carry on with what you're there for. This is the best way to portray a disciplined image and keep professional relationships strong.

Seek Support from Safe People

Knowing who "safe people" are is key in recovery. It's best to surround yourself with people who won't judge or criticize you. The safe people in your life could be your friends and family, or it could be a counselor if you feel you need a little more help than your personal circle of support can offer you.

Find support and seek comfort in people who know how to listen empathetically without feeling they need to say what they think you should do. Seek comfort in the people whom you know to have the ability to listen with compassion and have demonstrated kindness for the plight of others. Empathic listening skills may seem easy to find amongst friends and family, but this isn't always the case. Most people find it hard not to let preconceived notions or biases create judgments about people who are trying to recover from substance abuse. Most people would rather talk about what's interesting or beneficial for them. To be able to focus entirely on another person's life when there's nothing in it for you is a truly selfless act and far more difficult to master than basic listening skills. It requires you to walk a mile in the person's shoes by experiencing their emotions. You get to feel their happiness, sadness, anguish, joy, misery, and the challenges they face almost as though it was your journey. You'll often find that those who've suffered from addiction are the easiest to talk to.

It will take time to create your support system because building trust takes time. So, take the time to build your support team, and be sure you choose people who'll unselfishly support you and call you out when needed.

Chapter 9 – Sobriety Success

"Somebody once asked me how I define sobriety, and my response was 'liberation from dependence'." — Leslie Jamison

It's the moment you've long been waiting for, and you've marked this as the day of your rebirth. It's the beginning of a new life, new memories, and a new you. You've earned the right to celebrate it, go easy on yourself, and do the things you always wanted to do. Reaching success in sobriety means you're no longer a slave to alcohol. You've taken your power back, and your mind and body are finally under your command rather than your addiction controlling you.

Now that you've finally walked the long, winding road to the exit, you know, first-hand, how beautiful a sober life is. You see how much easier your life has become. You've seen friends coming back into your life, you're getting invited to events and social gatherings, and you're living life to the full. You no longer feel scared that alcohol will regain a hold on you, even in a situation where drinks are being pressed on you. You feel comfortable opting for an alcohol-free beverage.

Recognize that there's nothing wrong with needing to be alone sometimes, and you shouldn't feel guilty for giving yourself a treat every once in a while, either. It doesn't make you selfish to focus on yourself for a bit of time each day. You need that time to reorient your brain and stay strong in your recovery.

People often ask me whether sobriety can be long-term. People want to know if they can ever go back to the life they once had or have a drink every now and again. To this question specifically, I say this: "No, you can't go back to that life, and nor should you want to.

You left that life specifically because it was dangerous, destructive, and affected you negatively in countless ways."

Sobriety is a long-term decision. Here are some tips to help with your journey:
- Make time for recreation. While many people neglect this, you need this time. Find activities that you love or always wanted to try.
- Give yourself a spa day, and do it to the max.
- Keep a journal to reflect on how you feel.
- Stay in touch with your emotional and physical needs.
- Keep your treatment needs organized (using a calendar or other planning system) to ensure you take medications or attend sessions or appointments that will keep you strong and focused.
- Celebrate milestones by treating yourself to something nice. It always feels rewarding to save up a little money and give our self something special.

- Take time away from your devices because they can cause sleep problems and distract you from your needs.
- Learn how to appreciate the great outdoors. One of the best stress relievers is to spend time in Nature. The fresh air and the wonders of the Earth can revive your spirits. You don't need to spend a lot of time in Nature to start seeing the effects. Any place in Nature that you like will do. If you live in an urban area, finding a park or tending to houseplants or a community garden can be suitable options. Even just half an hour per day spent in the natural world can make you feel better, and you can combine your outdoor time with physical activity for additional benefits.
- Find films or podcasts on addiction and recovery so you can learn from the experiences and challenges of others and see how they were able to overcome even the most dire situations.

Now that you're on your way to recovering from this disorder don't lose track of the mental growth and discipline you've gained. Foster it with more knowledge by reading books on alcohol addiction.

Reading about what you've been through will remind you of your strength and perseverance each time you underestimate your potential. Stay in touch with people in your support groups, and volunteer to work to help others suffering from addiction. There's nothing more beautiful than meaningful work, and what better way to celebrate your success than by helping those who are going through what you've experienced. This is what will sustain your recovery for a lifetime.

Conclusion

"Everyone wants happiness. No one wants pain. But you can't have a rainbow without a little rain." – Anonymous

Alcoholism isn't a blame game. It isn't a choice you made but a disorder that consumed you. You're more than your addiction. You're much more than a slave to addictive urges. Millions are suffering from AUD, and many are in denial. Proclaiming, "No, I'm not an addict" is what mires sufferers deeper in their rut. What could be wonderful about losing control of your life to a bottle of liquor? Nothing. Alcohol has claimed many lives and is continuing to do so. This book attempts to provide insight into how to combat addiction starting with the first step—admitting you have a problem.

We all know alcohol is bad for the body and mind, but we tend to remain blind to this fact because the media and popular culture often portrays the abstainer as someone who's dull and lifeless. When a person in rehab is going through the devastating effects of withdrawal, they may be thinking how great it was to drink alcohol without feeling sick. The very acceptance of alcohol in our collective societies is at the core of the problem. This book is aimed not only at the AUD sufferer but anyone who might be contemplating drinking alcohol.

This book features to-the-point chapters describing the detrimental effects of drinking and supplements these with facts and figures compiled from empirical research in published journals. Some sections take a hard line with AUD, but sugar coating the repercussions of this complex disorder won't lead to a successful approach to recovery.

Lastly, this book encourages the reader to look at the brighter side of long-term recovery. An alcohol-free life is beautiful, and there are ways to deal with past pain and trauma that will eradicate them completely rather than drowning them for the moment in a glass. As you read through this book, you'll find yourself imagining a better version of yourself, with no secrets to keep and no dishonesty and shame to hide or answer for.

This book has a motivational theme that encourages zero tolerance for negative thoughts and emotions. It focuses on the biological aspects of AUD, its psychological basis, and the essentials of rehab. Mental health plays a fundamental role in recovery, and the road to sobriety incorporates a comprehensive approach. The topic of mental health is explored in an uncensored way, endorsing an ideology of acceptance of AUD to bring the much-awaited awareness to societies that tend to conceal or deny the reality of alcohol addiction. There's no shame in having AUD. It's not your fault, and yes, you can recover.

Sobriety is a long-term decision that I want each and every one of you reading this book to make. It might be frightening to hear you can't return to something that once gave you joy. I've discovered that the human mind tends to gloss over the bad parts of just about every experience in life. When we remember situations from ten years ago, it's easy to play down the negative elements. You'll be challenged throughout the coming years of your sobriety. Even when things are going well, your brain can cause you to second guess your decision-making abilities and make irrational choices. But don't worry. You aren't doomed!

I hope by now you know that long-term sobriety is the aim and bedrock of this book. Becoming sober means rebuilding your entire life so you don't find yourself in compromising situations or having to second-guess your decisions on a regular basis. Be strong, be confident, and enjoy your new-found life. Keep returning to this book when you need a refresher. Use it as a reference tool. And, if at any time you question anything you've read, feel free to send me an email.

I know you can do it.

One more thing

If you enjoyed this book and found it helpful, I'd be very grateful if you'd post a short review. Your support does make a difference, and I read all the reviews personally so I can get your feedback and make this book even better. I love hearing from my readers, and I'd really appreciate it if you leave your honest feedback.

Thank you for reading!

BONUS CHAPTER

I would like to share a sneak peek into another one of my books that I think you will enjoy. The book is titled **_"How to Deal with Stress, Depression, and Anxiety: A Vital Guide on How to Deal with Nerves and Coping with Stress, Pain, OCD, and Trauma."_**

Are you tired of wasting your time and energy worrying all the time? Do you see the irrationality of constant worrying, but you can't seem to stop doing it? Are you ready to learn how to deal with anxiety and depression without taking drugs?

This book will walk you through precisely why, how, and what you need to do to stop worrying and start living your life.

Nearly 800 million people worldwide experience mental illness. Some of the most prominent adverse mental conditions include stress, anxiety, and depression. These issues can affect your psychological and physical health, and when you let them go untreated, they can have longstanding effects on your life and relationships. The more you ignore your mental strife, the harder it becomes to be resilient in the face of hardship, and if you let emotions get out of hand, they can lead to increased mental illness.

Though stress is an inseparable part of our lives, we can easily manage it using simple strategies and techniques. All we need is the willingness to learn these techniques and the ability to take action. Effective stress management is critical to your physical, psychological, and emotional health. It's vital to your overall well-being. This book will show you how to start managing your issues and get relief immediately.

How to Deal with Stress, Depression, and Anxiety provides a complete framework and a well-rounded set of tools to understand the causes of stress, depression, anxiety and how to overcome it.

Enjoy this free chapter!

Virtually all people experience stress, anxiety, or depression at various points in their lives. One 2017 study suggested that about 792 million people worldwide have formal mental health disorders, with depression and anxiety being the most common conditions. Millions, maybe even billions, of additional people experience subclinical conditions and high levels of stress, so the number of people who deal daily with such issues is quite astounding. When you live with any of these conditions, everyday activities become a challenge, and you may resort to self-sabotaging behaviors, or you feel stuck in place.

As these conditions continue, it only makes you feel worse, both mentally and physically. In the United States, it's been reported that stress affects the mental health of 73 percent of the population, leading to worsening conditions like depression and anxiety. While these conditions are all too common, they don't have to be. Living with mental illness or stress can feel impossible, and that's a hard burden to carry, which is why mental distress often leads to further mental and emotional anguish.

The Challenge

With so much external pressure in today's society to be their best selves, millions of people worldwide struggle to maintain their mental health and professional or personal well-being. Many emotionally and physically harmful behaviors—such as overworking and extreme self-sacrifice—are glorified by society. As people are pushed to do their best work and make room for a personal and social life, they can become consumed by anxiety and worries that impede their progress.

The statistics on stress, anxiety, and depression depict a grim picture. As the most prevalent mental health issue in the United States, according to the Anxiety and Depression Association of America, anxiety impacts over 40 million American adults, representing over 18 percent of the population. Globally, nearly 300 million people have anxiety. People who have anxiety tend to have greater stress levels, and 50 percent of those diagnosed with anxiety will also be diagnosed with depression. Depression rates are also startlingly high, with just under seven percent of the population experiencing major depression at any given time and another two percent experiencing persistent depressive disorder, also known as dysthymia or chronic depression.

Even if you don't have a clinically diagnosed issue, such as depression or anxiety, you likely have some degree of stress that makes it harder to function as you'd like to. The Global Organization for Stress says that 75 percent of people are moderately stressed, and nearly all people experience stress at some point in their lives because of a myriad of contributing factors. With so much mental dysfunction, it's no wonder that some people think they'll never get better, but this grim picture doesn't have to be your reality.

While mental health conditions have the power to destroy and debilitate people—paralyzing them and making it hard to have hope for the future— there are proven techniques anyone can use to improve their mental health and allow greater opportunity for personal development. You do not need to let your stress, anxiety, or depression hold you back anymore.

The solution to managing your mental health isn't easy or quick, but it is effective. With effort and careful attention to a multi-faceted plan, you can make dramatic improvements to your damaged mental health and start investing more energy into things that make you the most gratified. There are several steps you must follow for the best results. When you apply these steps, you can have increased mental clarity, emotional freedom, and confidence. Curing your mental health issues will require you to face everything that scares you and to admit uncomfortable truths. Still, you'll be far better off when you seek help than the nearly 25 million Americans who have untreated mental health conditions. You may not need the same level of care as people with more severe conditions, but you do need help because living with any degree of stress, anxiety, or depression is living with more pain than you need to have.

Treating a mental illness can seem intimidating to many people, but there are several effective methods, and there are ways to treat, if not cure, any mental health condition you may have. With so many adults and children not currently being treated for their mental health issues, it's no wonder that mental health statistics remain so prevalent. Still, with increased awareness and the greater availability of mental health resources, the prognosis for those who have mental illness continues to improve. Alongside this, as these issues become more widely acknowledged and discussed, the stigmas attached to them are beginning to dissipate, which removes some of the shame linked to mental illness, which only exacerbates it. Accordingly, by committing bravely to treatment and opening yourself to increased understanding of mental illness, you create resilience against mental illness and become more proactive in the treatment of these debilitating conditions.

For those of you with any of these issues, you cannot delay treatment. Mental dysfunction of any kind makes it harder to feel joy and, in the worst cases, it can deprive you of your ability to function. More than that, your mental health can also impact your physical health. For example, research has shown that stress increases the chance of someone dying from cancer by 32 percent. The Canadian Mental Health Association says that people with poor mental health are more prone to having chronic physical disorders.

A study from Johns Hopkins University found that patients with a family history of heart disease were healthier when they engaged in positive thinking. Among the participants of the study, those who had a positive outlook were 13 percent less likely to experience a cardiac event. Additionally, they found that, generally, people who have better outlooks live longer.

The Solution

Recovery is a process that isn't always linear, but this book will lay out the basic steps to help get you on the right track. The first step in the process is all about education. Before you can do anything else, you must understand the beast you're trying to slaughter and the sword you'll use to slay it. You'll learn how the brain works and how problems with its wiring can lead to mental dysfunction. You'll also learn how you can rewire your cognitive processes to promote increased mental health.

In the second step of the process, you'll continue your educational journey and gain a more in-depth understanding of what anxiety, stress, and depression are and how they impact the way you function. You'll start to understand how to address each of these issues using essential coping tools.

Once you've learned about each condition, you'll be introduced to one of the most powerful psychological tools for improved mental health: Cognitive Behavioral Therapy (CBT). You'll discover what CBT is and how to use it to address your mental ailments.

Once you understand the founding principles of these conditions and the fundamentals of CBT, you'll learn how to manage your circumstances daily by overcoming roadblocks and reviving your sense of self by shifting your perspective as you begin to think in new ways. You'll start to care for both your body and your mind in life-changing ways. All of these steps will lead to mental clarity and mental liberation.

With all this in mind, it's clear that a person's mental health impacts every part of their life, and without addressing your mental dysfunction, you'll never have the peace of mind you crave. Each day you do nothing about your mental health is another day you deprive yourself of health and happiness. Your mental health should be your priority, because you cannot fully function as a member of society if you're prohibited from doing all the things you love the most.

If you feel like you are losing sight of yourself and your desires because of your stress, anxiety, or depression, it's time to make a change. It's okay to be nervous about the adjustments you will need to make to feel healthier, but remember that being uncomfortable and uncertain is vital because they represent change. If you don't change, you'll never feel better than you do now. Maybe you have learned to live with your pain and worry, but it's time to learn to live without those negative coping mechanisms because they stop you from living your life to the fullest.

While the techniques in this book can help you improve your levels of stress, anxiety, and depression, I recommend seeking professional support to help push you towards your goals.

There are tons of books on this subject on the market, so thank you for choosing this one! "How to Deal with

Stress, Depression, and Anxiety" will provide a complete framework and a well-rounded set of tools for you to understand the causes of stress, depression, anxiety and how to overcome it. Please enjoy!

How Your Brain Works

Too many people hurt their recovery journey by working against their minds. They think they can force their brains into submission, and when that doesn't work, they feel like failures. When a change you're trying to make doesn't stick, it is usually because it isn't one your brain is used to. As much as you may want that change, your brain will resist it because unfamiliar things feel unsafe to the human brain. The human brain loves patterns, and it uses those patterns to create your internal mental programming and perceptions of reality. When you understand how your brain works, you can use it to your advantage to create new patterns and reframe your mental state.

Your brain is a powerful force, and it can work in remarkable ways. In facing your worries, doubts, and other negative feelings, you need to understand how your brain functions so you can stop fighting your brain and start working with it.

Your Map of Reality

In 1931, scientist and philosopher Alfred Korzybski established an important metaphorical notion with his statement, "The map is not the territory." He believed that individuals don't have absolute knowledge of reality; instead, they have a set of beliefs built up over time that influence how they perceive events and situations. People's beliefs and views (their map) are not reality itself (the territory). In other words, perception is not reality.

Your brain fills gaps in understanding automatically. This means that when you don't know something, you subconsciously make an estimation based on the information you do know. When you experience worry or sadness, this can be caused by a map of reality that reinforces those ideas. That worry or sadness lingers in your mind and can shape future decisions unless you reshape your perception. Your map of reality will always be an interpretation, but it can be an interpretation that helps you rather than hurts you. You can change your map of reality and make it more productive by addressing your thoughts and beliefs and how they impact your behavior.

Thoughts, Core Beliefs, and Behavior
Beliefs are sets of ideas that individuals use to dictate

how they'll behave. A belief is something you think is a fact. You feel so strongly about something that you're almost positive it's true, regardless of how well you can prove it. You may have some doubts from time to time, but, overall, you consistently stick to those beliefs. Beliefs are attitudes that you fall back on, because they provide a sense of security, and they make you feel that certain things are constant, which is why something that makes you doubt your beliefs can be so painful. Your beliefs drive your unconscious, habitual behaviors. They become so ingrained in you that they feel natural and inherently true.

When you have trouble managing situations or coping with feelings, you automatically turn to your beliefs for help without exerting too much brainpower. Your beliefs help you determine morality, and they help you decide whether people or things are bad or good. Your whole perspective uses a compilation of your beliefs to fill in the parts of your reality you can't fully understand.

Beliefs are formed based on past experiences and the stimuli around us. Most people's core beliefs—the most driving beliefs they have—are established when they're young children. As they grow older, children commonly challenge the beliefs they've been taught as they begin to think more critically and independently. Nevertheless, many children reaffirm the beliefs they were taught rather than disproving them. As adults, they can challenge these beliefs and, by managing their beliefs, they can create a healthier view of the world that's a more realistic map of reality.

Beliefs can be incredibly powerful. For example, imagine parents telling their children that paperclips are dangerous. Telling a child that paperclips are dangerous seems silly. Nevertheless, when those words go unchallenged, the child will internalize the message, and they might try to avoid paperclips, which could impede their ability to do certain tasks. But as they grow older, the child would likely challenge that belief and overcome the fear of paperclips.

Other beliefs may be harder to debunk. For instance, if a mom tells her child that dogs are dangerous, the child may become afraid of dogs. This fear could continue into adulthood, because the child has learned to be terrified of dogs. Even rational arguments that dogs aren't something to be scared of may still make it hard for that child to believe. After all, dogs, unlike paperclips, do have the potential to bark and bite. The child would be so convinced by the belief that it would be hard for them to break from that mindset.

You may have beliefs that stand in your way and feel so foundational to who you are that challenging them makes you uncomfortable. Nevertheless, you need to contemplate your limiting beliefs.

While thoughts and beliefs may seem similar, there are some profound differences between them that you must acknowledge if you want to have a complete understanding of how your thoughts and beliefs can make or break your mental health. Thoughts help to form your beliefs. When you have the same thoughts repeatedly, they become beliefs. You become so used to the thoughts that they become ingrained in your subconscious, and it becomes hard to imagine that those thoughts aren't true. Accordingly, when you think negatively, you tend to have a more pessimistic outlook.

Not all thoughts are beliefs. The thoughts that come and go through your mind without repetition never become beliefs. Beliefs are a product of habitual thinking. This means that while it may be hard to break them, you can break them by overwriting those negative thoughts with positive ones, which is a practice that many therapies and techniques discussed in this book use to reduce stress, anxiety, and depression.

As you've seen with the map of reality, perception shapes our views, and it also shapes the way we think. Your thoughts build your beliefs, and your beliefs, in turn, build your sense of what's real. Some of your beliefs will empower you to seek success and find happiness, while others will make the world seem like a dark and scary place with no hope. Try to identify the parts of your belief system that cause you to have negative responses.

Your thought patterns have tremendous power to change your life. The simple act of interrupting negative thought patterns can help you begin to make changes. These changes don't happen overnight, and deeply entrenched beliefs may even take months or years to debunk completely, but, when you focus on the thought patterns you want to instill, you start to question the "truths" you blindly believed.

There will be some beliefs you'll want to keep, and those are ones you can build upon and use to your advantage throughout this process. There's no need to get rid of any belief that's constructive because such beliefs are the ones that help you grow. However, be honest about the beliefs that are hurting you. Many people try to rationalize certain beliefs that they feel psychologically unready to call into question. Open your mind and contemplate, "Is this belief hurting me in covert and manipulative ways?" If you struggle even to pose that question about a particular belief, that belief may be a harmful one.

The way you think isn't something that's out of your control. According to the Massachusetts Institute of Technology (MIT), 45 percent of your daily choices are habitual, meaning they're a product of your subconscious thought patterns and beliefs. You choose what stimuli you feed to your subconscious. When worries or hopelessness begin to fill your head, try saying to yourself, "The world is a place full of opportunity and good things." While it won't feel like saying this is doing anything at first, rewriting your internal monologue can be a powerful first step toward growth.

When you understand how thoughts and core beliefs shape your behaviors, it becomes easier to create a path for growth. You learn that you're in charge of your beliefs, and your thoughts can only have as much control over you as you give them. You may feel helpless against your negative thoughts, but learning to overcome these harmful thoughts and release the power they have over you is the only way to become a happier person. The more you try to avoid the things that make you anxious, stressed, or depressed, the more anxious, stressed, and depressed you'll become.

Cognitive Distortions

While your brain does its best to give you helpful information and create an accurate perception of reality, sometimes it gets a little lost trying to translate what it observes into a sensible perception. Your brain loves to make connections, and sometimes, it will make connections that are overly simplified and don't show the nuance in a situation. This is called a cognitive distortion.

Simple speaking, cognitive distortions are falsehoods that your brain persuades you into believing are true. Cognitive distortions can take a variety of forms, but one common example is polarized thinking. When you think in polarities, you see things as wrong or right, good or bad, or win or lose. After you fail at one task, you may start to think, "I'll fail every task because I can't do anything right." This perception isn't an accurate one, but you become convinced it's true because your brain has pinpointed what it thinks is a pattern.

The problem with cognitive distortions is that they're often shrouded in negativity. They make you expect the worse, and they convince you that you cannot do certain things or that other things are unsafe. Cognitive distortions change your perspective, and they can quickly become harmful to your overall well-being. If you believe false messages, it's hard to make peace with your situation or feel secure. When you feel insecure, your mental health declines, and your doubts start to make it harder to function normally. Anxiety may take hold, and you may feel more stressed as you try to complete tasks. The hardship of your situation may then lead to depression.

Cognitive distortions can also cause you to act in ways that worsen your mental state. For example, someone with an eating disorder may tell themselves, "Not eating helps me," when they lose a couple of pounds. They keep going with harmful behaviors because a faulty pattern was established of believing that an action is "good," even though the behavior, for obvious reasons, is the opposite of helpful.

Likewise, someone with anxiety may say, "Avoiding this task will make me feel calmer," when procrastination only heaps on the pressure and stress of the situation. Delaying the task may have given them a sense of relief before, so they keep doing it. It continues to impair them, but cognitive distortion causes them to keep repeating the same harmful behavior. Cognitive distortions fool you into thinking certain actions are good for you or that they aren't as harmful as they are. Someone may engage in risky behavior and think, "This won't hurt me because it didn't harm me before," when that's not accurate information. People often use these distortions to justify harmful, habitual behaviors that give temporary relief to mental distress, but this causes more problems in the long run.

Negative Thoughts

Negative thoughts can play an influential role in how your brain works because your thoughts help create your map of reality and form your cognitive distortions. It's much easier to give in to negative thoughts than positive ones. People often expect the worst because they're afraid that having hope will lead to disappointment. Negative thoughts are also fueled by the internalization of negative comments that others have made about you in the past. For instance, if your mother tells you that you're ugly, you may start to think you're unattractive until it ultimately becomes a core belief.

Research has shown how much healthier and happier

people are when they think positively because the brain responds to the input we give it. So, you can change your outlook by thinking with more positivity. When you think negatively, you're feeding your brain with information it can use against you; therefore, give it information that will help you instead!

<u>The Role of Trauma</u>
Trauma is a significant part of human life, and it can be one of the largest contributors to adverse mental health outcomes, including increased depression, anxiety, and stress. According to the National Council for Behavioral Health, 70 percent of adults in the United States have experienced at least one traumatic event, which means that 223.4 million people in the United States alone have had trauma. Moreover, among people who seek treatment for mental health issues, 90 percent have gone through trauma. Consequently, if you have trauma, it contributes to some of the issues you may be experiencing.

Trauma is the result of events that cause deep worry or distress. Traumatic experiences are often those that either threaten a person's life or the life or well-being of those they love.

You can have both physical and emotional trauma. Physical trauma can be a response to accidents, injuries, or other physical events. Physical trauma often can trigger emotional trauma, and the scars from emotional trauma often linger longer than those of physical trauma. Trauma can result from physical, verbal, emotional, or sexual abuse, and children who live in violent environments are at an increased risk for trauma. Some people don't realize they have trauma. They might say, "Oh, well, what I went through wasn't that bad compared to other people." However, trauma doesn't mean you were tortured or injured in unthinkable ways. The death of people you love or contracting a serious disease can also cause trauma. Anything can be traumatic if it makes you feel unsafe, so don't downplay those feelings—accept how you feel, even if you don't think it's "that bad."

When you have trauma that you haven't addressed, you're bound to have increased mental challenges. Trauma alone doesn't lead to mental illness, but it's a major contributing factor, and it drives you to rely on unhealthy coping mechanisms that do you more harm than good.

Trauma changes the way you think, which can impact your decision-making processes and your unconscious thoughts. Trauma makes your brain feel unsafe, and when your brain feels unsafe, it focuses on protecting you from future pain, because that pain could threaten your survival. Even in circumstances that don't usually cause anxiety, you may start to feel threatened, even if you can't logically explain why. When you go through trauma, your brain has a stress response, and that stress response reacts to the trauma by changing your future behaviors in an attempt to protect you.

The stress response involves areas of the brain, including the prefrontal cortex, hippocampus, and amygdala. These areas experience lingering changes when they undergo the intense pressure of trauma. As a result, the way your brain processes information shifts when you experience trauma. Your amygdala becomes more active. This part of your brain is responsible for your flight-or-fight reactions and, when it's overactive, it can make you feel as though you're in danger in non-dangerous situations. It stays on guard because it wants to prevent any potential threats from sneaking up on you.

When your amygdala becomes more active, you may be more prone to feeling stressed, and the hippocampus—the part of your brain that handles short-term memories—may become less active. As a result, you may struggle to differentiate between things that happened to you in the past and things that are presently happening.

Finally, the pre-cortex may shrink, and when it does, you have trouble dealing with your emotions and regulating your thoughts. Many of these changes can be found in people who have post-traumatic stress disorder (PTSD), but anyone with trauma can experience them to a lesser degree.

For obvious reasons, trauma makes it hard for you to be mentally healthy, but it also makes it hard for you to be physically healthy. When your physical health declines, this creates additional causes of anxiety, stress, and depression. Thus, not only can your mental health make your physical health worse, but your physical health can make your mental health worse. The Canadian Mental Health Association reports that people with depression are three times as likely to have chronic pain than people without depression. People who have chronic pain are two times as likely to have anxiety or a mood disorder. Mental and physical health are often dependent on one another, which is why the correlations between the two are so important.

According to statistics, you are more likely to experience health issues such as chronic obstructive pulmonary disease (COPD), heart disease, high blood pressure, cancer, and diabetes when you have trauma. These conditions can all reduce your life's quality or longevity, which can then create even more mental unrest. That psychological turbulence can lead to your physical conditions worsening. You can see how these situations can quickly become bleak for those experiencing them. However, by addressing your trauma, you can reduce the potency of some of these issues.

Trauma, unfortunately, is a normal part of life. For

many people, it's challenging to manage, but it's nothing to be ashamed of. Using the strategies in this book, you can learn to become conscious of your trauma and take away the power it has to control your life. Simple techniques like listening to music, establishing a healthy diet and exercise routine, practicing meditation, and admitting you have trauma are just some of the most basic techniques you can use to recover.

Recovery from trauma is painful, but it's one of the most important things you can do for your health because working through trauma allows you to heal your brain and teach it new patterns.

Get Professional Help

Before you do anything, you should seek professional help. Seeing a doctor or a mental health professional can help ensure that you have a support system in place to help you improve yourself.

While this book's techniques can help you improve your levels of stress, anxiety, and depression, some people will still need professional support to help push them toward their goals. Additionally, for some people, these issues may be related to their brain chemistry, which may require medication. To have a satisfactory recovery experience, you must take a holistic approach that ensures you achieve long-lasting results and can learn coping skills that will shape the rest of your life.

Get your full copy today! ***"How to Deal with Stress, Depression, and Anxiety: A Vital Guide on How to Deal with Nerves and Coping with Stress, Pain, OCD, and Trauma."***

BOOKS BY RICHARD BANKS

How to be Charismatic, Develop Confidence, and Exude Leadership: The Miracle Formula for Magnetic Charisma, Defeating Anxiety, and Winning at Communication

How to Stop Being Negative, Angry, and Mean: Master Your Mind and Take Control of Your Life

How to Deal with Grief, Loss, and Death: A Survivor's Guide to Coping with Pain and Trauma, and Learning to Live Again

How to Deal With Stress, Depression, and Anxiety: A Vital Guide on How to Deal with Nerves and Coping with Stress, Pain, OCD and Trauma

The Positive Guide to Anger Management: The Most Practical Guide on How to Be Calmer, Learn to Defeat Anger, Deal with Angry People, and Living a Life of

Mental Wellness and Positivity

Develop a Positive Mindset and Attract the Life of Your Dreams: Unleash Positive Thinking to Achieve Unbound Happiness, Health, and Success

The Keys to Being Brilliantly Confident and More Assertive: A Vital Guide to Enhancing Your Communication Skills, Getting Rid of Anxiety, and Building Assertiveness

Personal Development Mastery 2 Books in 1: The Keys to being Brilliantly Confident and More Assertive + How to be Charismatic, Develop Confidence, and Exude Leadership

Positive Mindset Mastery 2 Books in 1: Develop a Positive Mindset and Attract the Life of Your Dreams + How to Stop Being Negative, Angry, and Mean

Printed in Dunstable, United Kingdom